Living with
renal failure

Living with renal failure

Proceedings of a Multidisciplinary Symposium
held at the University of Stirling, 7–8 July, 1977

Edited by
J. L. Anderton
Consultant Renal Physician, Western General
Hospital, Edinburgh
F. M. Parsons
Consultant Nephrologist, General Infirmary,
Leeds
D. E. Jones
Nursing Officer, Renal Unit, St. Bartholomew's
and St. Leonard's Hospitals, London

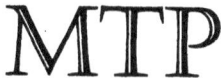

Published by
MTP Press Limited
St. Leonard's House
Lancaster, England

ISBN-13: 978-94-011-6187-9   e-ISBN-13: 978-94-011-6185-5
DOI: 10.1007/978-94-011-6185-5

Contents

SECTION THREE

Some Clinical Problems
Chairman: J. S. Cameron

SECTION FOUR

Psychological and Personal Aspects
Chairman: M. Carmody

SECTION FIVE

Practical Management
Chairman: A. C. Kennedy

List of Contributors

Dr J. L. ANDERTON
Consultant Physician in Renal Diseases, Nuffield Transplant Unit, Western General Hospital, Edinburgh

Mr J. BAILLIE
Director, Tullis Neill Limited, Mayfield, Dalkeith, Edinburgh

Dr J. D. BRIGGS
Consultant Physician in Renal Diseases, Western Infirmary, Glasgow

Mrs MARY BROWN
Home Dialysis Sister, Renal Transplant and Dialysis Unit, Manchester Royal Infirmary, Manchester

Professor J. S. CAMERON
Professor in Renal Medicine, Guy's Hospital, London

Dr M. CARMODY
Consultant Nephrologist, St. Mary's Hospital, Dublin

Dr W. R. CATTELL
Consultant Nephrologist, St. Bartholomew's Hospital, London

Dr T. G. FEEST
Senior Registrar, Royal Victoria Infirmary, Newcastle-upon-Tyne

Mrs JEAN K. GIBBINS
Renal Unit, Royal Infirmary, Sunderland

Mr D. N. H. HAMILTON
Lecturer in Surgery, Western Infirmary, Glasgow

Dr J. A. HENRY
Senior Registrar, Department of Medicine, University College Hospital, London

Dr D. S. JAMES
Department of Child and Family Psychiatry, Royal Hospital for Sick Children, Glasgow

Mrs DEIRDRE E. JONES
Nursing Officer, Renal Unit, St. Bartholomew's and St. Leonard's Hospitals, London

Mr A. McL. JENKINS
Senior Lecturer in Surgery, Royal Infirmary, Edinburgh

Dr J. A. KANIS
Wellcome Senior Clinical Research Fellow, Renal Unit, The Churchill Hospital, Oxford

Professor A. C. KENNEDY
University Department of Medicine, Royal Infirmary, Glasgow

Miss KIRSTY M. MARSHALL
Senior Fieldwork Teacher, Training and Development, Social Work Headquarters, Lothian Region, Edinburgh

Dr A. M. MARTIN
Consultant Physician, Renal Unit, Royal Infirmary, Sunderland

Miss KATHLEEN NICHOLSON
Nursing Officer, Renal Unit, Western Infirmary, Glasgow

Dr D. M. PARKIN
Community Physician, Leeds Area Health Authority, Leeds

Dr F. M. PARSONS
Consultant in Clinical Renal Physiology, The General Infirmary, Leeds

Dr B. H. B. ROBINSON
Consultant Physician, Department of Renal Medicine, East Birmingham Hospital, Birmingham

Professor J. S. ROBSON
Professor of Medicine, The University of Edinburgh and Director of the Medical Renal Unit at the Royal Infirmary, Edinburgh

Miss HELEN ROSENTHAL
Home Dialysis Administrator, St. Leonard's/St. Bartholomew's Regional Renal Unit, London

Dr A. W. SIEMSEN
Director, Institute of Renal Diseases, Saint Francis Hospital, Honolulu, Hawaii

Miss SALLY TABER
Nursing Officer, Professorial Unit, Addenbrookes Hospital, Cambridge

Dr T. WALMSLEY
Dept. of Psychiatry, Royal Infirmary, Edinburgh

Dr M. K. WARD
Lecturer in Medicine, University of Newcastle-upon-Tyne

Dr R. J. WINNEY
Senior Registrar, Medical Renal Unit, (University of Edinburgh), The Royal Infirmary, Edinburgh

Preface

The management of chronic renal failure by dialysis and transplantation has now become an established form of treatment in many parts of the world. However, these forms of treatment have brought with them problems in relation to the selection of patients, economics, clinical problems such as hypertension, encephalopathy, anaemia and renal bone disease, and psychological and social problems. The management of haemodialysis has changed over the years with developments in dialysers, vascular access and the duration of dialysis. Although the overall survival from renal transplantation has changed little in the past four or five years, there are hopes of improvements in relation to tissue typing and enhancement.

Perhaps the most important aspect in the management of chronic renal failure is the multi-disciplinary approach. Nursing and medical staff work closely with dialysis technicians, engineers, dietitians, local authority personnel, social workers and with the relatives of the patients.

The symposium was planned to draw together representatives from all disciplines involved in the care of patients with chronic renal failure. One of the most relevant sessions was that in which two patients with chronic renal failure described their experience.

Travenol Laboratories Limited sponsored the symposium and provided the administrative services. The contributors and editors are deeply grateful for the opportunity that this has given them to reach a wider public with a message whose importance grows daily. The editors acknowledge the helpful collaboration of our publisher and the skill of Mrs Judy Fagleston who transcribed the discussions. Finally, they wish to thank Peter Irving of Travenol Laboratories who organized the symposium and who enabled us all to respond to the challenge of "Living with Renal Failure".

JLA
FMP
DEJ

Introduction
F. M. Parsons

Two hundred years ago Cotunnius[1] associated oedema with coagulable substances in the urine. These observations were brilliantly extended by Richard Bright 50 years later[2] who, in collaboration with his chemist Dr Bostock, demonstrated a disturbance in excretion of urea associated with a full pulse, oedema, albuminous urine and contracted kidneys. One year later, in 1828, Wohler was the first to synthesize urea from inorganic radicles and wrote to Berzelius: 'I must tell you that I can prepare urea without requiring a kidney or an animal, either man or dog'[3].

In 1832 another landmark occurred. Thomas Thompson, Professor of Chemistry, University of Glasgow, who was also medically qualified, investigated the biochemical imbalance produced by malignant cholera[4], which was then endemic in the United Kingdom. Dr O'Shaughnessy[5] both extended and reported Professor Thompson's work in the *Lancet* and concluded that salts and water left the blood to enter the rice stools. Dr Latta, a clinician from Leith who probably worked in the Drummond Street Cholera Hospital, Edinburgh (situated close to the Old Royal Infirmary), logically interpreted the data of Thompson and O'Shaughnessy with amazing insight for that era and 'resolved to throw the fluid immediately into the circulation'[6] in extreme cases when the deficit could not be corrected via the gastrointestinal tract. Dr Latta recorded several examples of the beneficial use of intravenous therapy in his report to the Central Board of Health, London[6]. It would appear that he suffered the fate that many pioneers of newer forms of successful therapy encounter. In the management of one patient found *in extremis* and given intravenous fluid in her home he recorded[7]: 'A female, aged 50, very destitute, but previously in good health, was on the 13th instant, at four a.m., seized with cholera in its most violent form, and by half-past nine was reduced to a most hopeless state. The pulse was quite gone, even in the axilla, and strength so much exhausted, that I had resolved not to try the effects of the injection, conceiving the poor woman's case to be hopeless, and that the failure of the experiment might afford the prejudiced and the illiberal an opportunity to stigmatize the practice; however, I at length thought I would give her a chance, and in the presence of Drs Lewins and Craigie, and Messrs. Sibson and Paterson, I injected one hundred and twenty ounces, when like the effects of magic, instead of the pallid aspect of one whom death had sealed as his own, the vital tide was restored, and life and vivacity returned'.

Presumably Messrs Sibson and Paterson were solicitors and had been asked to attend as independent witnesses to this very new and controversial therapy. The patient made an excellent recovery and was then 'for better accommodation, carried to the hospital'. In 1832 this must have been considered a highly scientific exercise based, as it was, on an accurate assessment of the biochemical abnormality induced by cholera and exhibited all the criteria of correct fluid and electrolyte therapy as used today.

Dr Craigie, a colleague of Dr Latta, recorded the treatment of another patient[7]. 'Martha Smith, aged 38, a noted drunkard, thin and debilitated in sixth month of pregnancy, admitted into the hospital at 8 p.m., May 16th, 1832'. She was treated conventionally with 'saline' enemas but at 11.30 a.m. the findings were: 'Breathing becoming much affected; extreme restlessness; cramps severe in legs, and every symptom of sinking. Let the following saline solution be injected into one of the veins of the arm.

> ℞   *Muriat. sodæ* ʒi ;
>   *Carbon. sodæ* gr. **x** ;
>   *Aq. calid.* ℔iiij, *solve temp.* **105°**
>   *Fahr.*

Noon. When about ℔i [i.e. about 450 ml] had been thrown in, the pulse was perceived to flutter at the wrist, and gradually strengthened as the injection was proceeded with. By the time ℔iiiss [i.e. about 1.5 l] had been injected, the countenance, which was before quite death-like, now beamed with the appearance of health, and she began to converse freely. Pulse 96, moderate. To have ʒi gin in warm water with sugar.

Half-past one. The gin was immediately rejected'.

She required two further intravenous injections, making a total of about 4 litres in all, and then Dr Craigie reported: 'Has passed about ℔j [i.e. about 450 ml] of urine, of natural appearance; this is the first she has made since she was brought in'.

The composition of the fluid given intravenously was $NaCl$ 45.0 mEq/l and $NaHCO_3$ 5.3 mEq/l. Thus, these accounts of the world's first intravenous fluid therapy also include the first known correction of a pre-renal failure.

In 1830 Thomas Graham (Figure 1), a Scot, was appointed to the first independent chair of chemistry at Anderson's University, Glasgow. He moved to University College, London, in 1837 and became Warden and Master Worker of the Mint in 1855[8]. Graham was one of the great scientists of the nineteenth century (see Graham's Law on the Diffusion of Gases) but to nephrologists he will be remembered for his experiments with

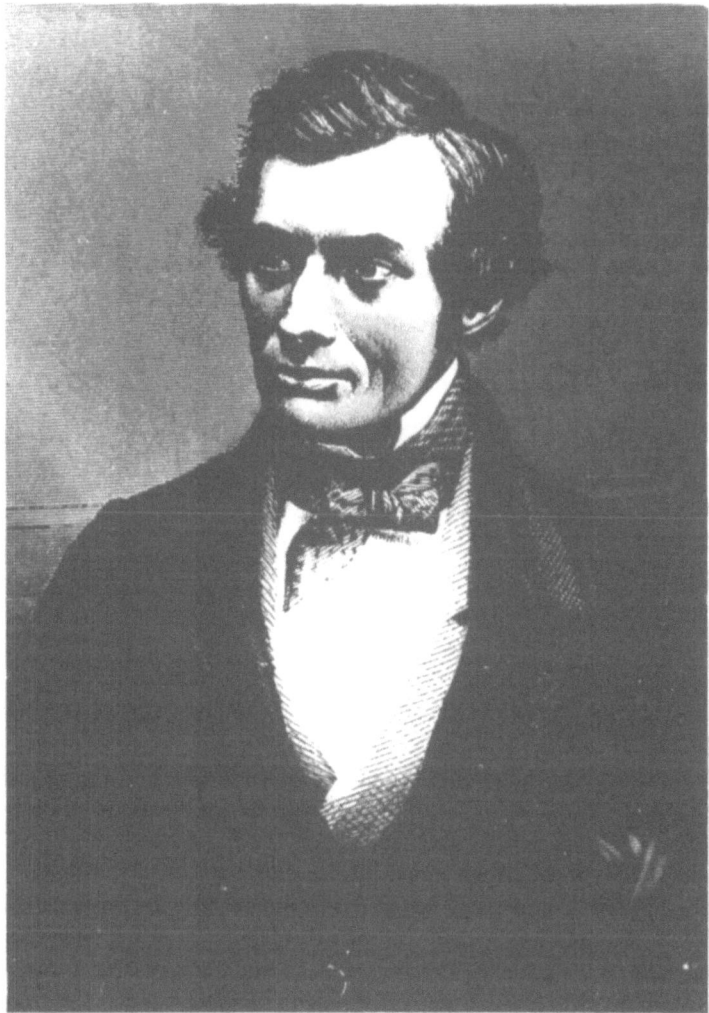

Figure 1   Thomas Graham (1805–69)

the membrane parchment (manufactured by the firm of Messrs De la Rue) which he attached to a wooden or (preferably) a guttapercha hoop (Figure 2) which was then floated on water – the 'Graham hoop dialyser'[9]. He demonstrated that when colloids and crystalloids were placed in the hoop only crystalloids passed through to enter the water. He coined the phrase 'dialysis' (from the Greek *dia*, through and *luein*, to loosen) to describe the

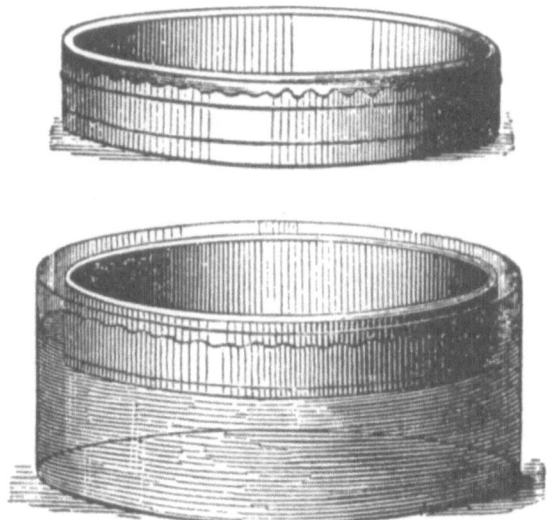

Figure 2   The Graham hoop dialyser

process. He used his 'dialyser' for much experimental work on crystalloids and colloids.

It was not until 1912 that haemodialysis was used experimentally on the dog by Abel, Rowntree and Turner[10]. This dialyser, which used celloidin as a semipermeable membrane and hirudin as an anticoagulant, was further developed by Haas in Germany[11] who was the first person to perform haemodialysis on the human. Technical problems, though, were plentiful.

In the 1940s four groups took up the challenge, each working independently. Kolff[12] must take the initial honours with the design and development of the rotating drum artificial kidney but the valuable contributions made by Alwall[13], Murray *et al.*[14] and Skeggs and Leonards[15] cannot be ignored. By the early 1950s haemodialysis was well established for the management of patients with reversible types of renal failure and in 1956 the first artificial kidney unit in the United Kingdom was opened in the General Infirmary at Leeds. Treatment then settled down to a relatively quiet peaceful routine until the development of the Scribner Shunt in 1960[16]. Overnight the scene changed, for in this single, but simple, breakthrough the long-term management of patients with irreversible types of renal failure became possible. It must be remembered, though, that it had taken over 200 years of progressive endeavour by scientists and physicians to achieve this desirable goal.

As the life of patients with terminal renal failure has now been usefully extended by intermittent dialysis new problems have inevitably emerged and many of these will be discussed during this symposium. Pre-existing disease processes have become exacerbated. New syndromes have developed whilst technical problems have been lessened or even solved. What are the inner thoughts of patients who spend many hours strapped to a machine? Is it a bearable life? Is transplantation desired by patients? What are the social and economic implications? For we are all too conscious that none could afford therapy without financial help from the community.

Speakers have been chosen to introduce these and other topics but it is hoped that everyone will join in the subsequent discussions.

ACKNOWLEDGEMENTS

Figure 1 was kindly supplied by Edith Frame, Sub-Librarian, University of Strathclyde.

Figure 2 is reproduced by permission of the Librarian of the Royal Society and the quotations are reprinted by permission of the Editor of the *Lancet*.

References

1. Robson, J. S. (1967). The nephrotic syndrome. In D. A. K. Black (ed.). *Renal Disease*, pp. 275–308. (Oxford: Blackwell Scientific Publications)
2. Bright, R. (1827). *Reports of Medical Cases*, Vol 1 (London: Longmans Green)
3. Feiser, L. F. and Feiser, M. (1961). *Advanced Organic Chemistry*, p. 3. (New York: Rheinhold Publishing Corporation)
4. Thompson, T. (1832). Chemical Analysis of the Blood of Cholera Patients. *Philosophical Magazine and Annals*, 11, 345
5. O'Shaughnessy, W. B. (1832). Chemical pathology of cholera. *Lancet*, ii, 225
6. Latta, T. (1832). Documents communicated by the Central Board of Health, London, relative to the treatment of cholera by the copious injection of aqueous and saline fluids into the veins. *Lancet*, ii, 274
7. Craigie, T. (1832). Details of two cases of malignant cholera treated by venous injection. *Lancet*, ii, 277
8. Frame, E. (1970). Thomas Graham: A Centenary Account. *Trans. R. Soc. Glasgow*, 7, 116
9. Graham, T. (1861). Liquid diffusion applied to analysis. *Phil. Trans. R. Soc.*, 151, 183
10. Abel, J. J., Rowntree, L. G. and Turner, B. B. (1913). Some constituents of the blood. *J. pharmacol. exp. ther.*, 5, 611
11. Drukker, W. (1978). Haemodialysis—A Historical Review. In W. Drukker,

F. M. Parsons and J. Maher (eds.). *Replacement of Renal Function by Dialysis.* (The Hague: Martinus Nijhoff, B. V.) (in press)

12. Kolff, W. J. (1947). *New Ways of Treating Uraemia.* (London: J. & A. Churchill)

13. Alwall, N. (1947). On the artificial kidney. I. Apparatus for dialysis of the blood *in vivo. Acta Med. Scand.,* **128,** 317

14. Murray, G., Delorme, E. and Thomas, N. (1947). Development of an artificial kidney. *Arch. Surg.,* **55,** 505

15. Skeggs, L. T. and Leonards, J. R. (1948). Studies on an artificial kidney. I. Preliminary results with a new type of continuous dialyzer. *Science,* **108,** 212

16. Scribner, B. H., Hegstrom, R. M. and Buri, R. (1961). Treatment of chronic uremia by means of hemodialysis: a progress report. In G. Richet (ed.) *First International Congress of Nephrology,* p. 616. (Basle: S. Karger AG)

SECTION ONE

Meeting the Needs
Chairman:
J. S. Robson

1

Selection of patients for dialysis and transplantation
B. H. B. Robinson

1.1   EARLY DEVELOPMENTS AND SELECTION

The success of Scribner's group in Seattle, in overcoming the problem of repeated vascular access for haemodialysis and making possible regular dialysis for chronic renal failure[1], came not only as an exciting new venture for nephrologists but as a challenge for those who have to decide financing and priorities in health care. The inevitable and unpleasant death in uraemia for those in chronic renal failure was averted and the patients returned to active life. It soon became clear that regular dialysis therapy would pose many problems. These were economic and political on the one hand – for here was a dramatic and effective treatment for an inevitably fatal disease, but a very expensive treatment – and medical on the other. Which patients would prove most suitable for therapy and rehabilitation? What complications were to be expected? The latter question was answered in part after only a few years, as renal bone disease, ectopic calcification, neuropathy and dialysis-associated hepatitis began to appear.

At the same time as regular dialysis treatment (RDT) was being developed, new progress was made in renal transplantation by the application of relatively safer and more effective immunosuppressive regimens. At first, dialysers and transplanters seemed to be apparently in competition, but during the past decade have worked in very close cooperation in offering an improved outlook for patients with chronic renal disease. The relative indications for treatment have changed as facilities have become more generally available. The economic aspects of treatment are to be dealt with in a later session, but with our present dearth of facilities medical criteria will be important in determining priorities.

In many western countries facilities have been developed to treat all subjects with end-stage renal failure, and selection is a thing of the past. Some of us are less fortunate[2]. After a promising start in the UK the lack of any politically or administratively directed policy from the centre, as much as economic stringency, has resulted in a considerable shortfall of treatment facilities, despite the urgings of nephrologists.

I propose to examine the various factors which we have to consider when a patient presents in advanced renal failure, and discuss the way in which these factors affect suitability for treatment and the method of treatment chosen.

1.2 TYPE OF PRIMARY RENAL DISEASE AND SELECTION

Dialysis treatment was initially confined to patients with uncomplicated renal disease. Those with systemic disease such as amyloidosis and diabetes were excluded. Patients in the former group still constitute the vast majority undergoing treatment. The largest single diagnostic group of patients is included in the miscellaneous classification of glomerulonephritis, with pyelonephritis and the various forms of interstitial nephritis second. Polycystic disease and primary hypertension account for large minority groups. The influence of hypertension upon selection will be discussed below. Several reports have emphasized the exceptionally good results obtained with RDT in the treatment of patients with polycystic disease. Their prognosis and rehabilitation are better than average, and most patients have normal or near normal haematocrits in happy contrast with most of their fellows. European experience[3] suggests that results in polycystic disease are less impressive for renal transplantation, results being similar or even a little worse in age-matched controls with other renal disorders.

One might suppose that some forms of glomerulonephritis, particularly those in which an active immunopathogenic mechanism is strongly suspect, would recur in transplanted kidneys, yet no consistent pattern has been reported even for rapidly progressive glomerulonephritis[4]. In 300 transplants we have seen recurrences of crescentic glomerulonephritis in only two, leading to graft failure after 6 and 8 months respectively. In several other patients it has not been possible to distinguish between recurrent glomerulonephritis and chronic rejection. Early and severe recurrence of focal glomerulosclerosis (FGS) has been reported in allografts[5]. In our limited experience with transplantation in this condition we have seen one patient in whom heavy proteinuria led to a nephrotic syndrome within a month of grafting but in another similar patient there has been no recurrence after 18 months. Recurrence has not been universal[4,6] and this diagnosis need not debar at least one attempt at transplantation. Although the histological changes of membrano-proliferative with dense deposits may recur in allografts[4], the clinical significance of this is not yet apparent.

Thus it seems that with the possible exception of FGS, which may sometimes recur in the transplant, the initiating renal disorder *per se* has little influence on selection, and little or no influence on selection as between dialysis or transplantation, although massive polycystic kidneys, recurrent infection or an abnormal lower urinary tract may require preliminary surgery. A bladder severely affected by tuberculosis or other pathology may bias one in favour of dialysis, although the ureter may be implanted into an ileal-loop conduit.

Analgesic nephropathy has been considered a relative contraindication in some centres because it suggests a personality disorder in the individual. In practice we have found that these patients do well on dialysis. One patient, having given up his analgesics, recovered sufficient renal function after five months RDT to be taken off the programme and to survive in comparatively good health on mild protein restriction alone, until he died 20 months later following a myocardial infarction. A few patients unfortunately continue to take analgesics after transplantation, and may endanger their graft. There is also an increased risk of carcinoma of the renal pelvis in this condition[7], and we have lost one dialysis patient from this cause.

1.3 HYPERTENSION AND CARDIOVASCULAR PROBLEMS IN SELECTION

Hypertension has been present in more than half the patients we have accepted for the dialysis programme and in 15% has been in the accelerated (malignant) phase. Hypertension has been easily controlled by dialysis in nearly all patients. We have found bilateral nephrectomy necessary only for dialysis-resistant hypertension with grossly elevated plasma renin levels in three patients out of nearly 500 entering our combined programme. Several other patients have had a bilateral nephrectomy with only moderate effect on the hypertension. These proved to be individuals who abused fluid restriction. These patients can be a serious problem in a dialysis unit but they are not easy to identify before starting therapy.

Diazoxide is a valuable drug for reducing the very high blood pressure of malignant hypertension, and minoxidil is of value in the resistant blood pressure associated with chronic renal failure. More recent experience with diafiltration suggests that we may have another valuable tool[8].

Hypertension is often a complication of chronic renal disease and, unless prolonged, has not significantly altered prognosis in our group, although most, but not all, deaths from cerebral infarction or haemorrhage have been in patients previously hypertensive. Prognostically, a large heart and angina have been unfavourable selection criteria. None of our patients starting dialysis with angina have survived 5 years. But care must be taken to distinguish angina from the pain and apparent cardiomegaly of uraemic pericarditis, for this condition is responsive to dialysis – although initially we prefer peritoneal dialysis to diminish the risk of haemorrhagic effusion and tamponade. If we have selected a patient for dialysis we endeavour to commence therapy before pericarditis develops.

Few would plan dialysis or transplantation for those who have had severe strokes but limited experience of patients who have had transient ischaemic attacks or even a minor, largely recovered, hemiparesis has been encouraging. Nevertheless myocardial infarction and cerebral vascular accidents are major causes of late mortality in dialysis and transplantation[3]. Perhaps we should pay more attention to the hyperlipidaemia which is so common in uraemic subjects.

Peripheral vascular disease may be so severe as to make vascular access for dialysis almost impossible, even with newer techniques for grafting vascular prosthesis (bovine carotid, umbilical vein or expanded polytetrafluoroethylene (PTFE). Vascular calcification associated with hyperparathyroidism is an important factor in many patients, and another indication for early management of uraemia and avoidance of overenthusiastic vitamin D therapy.

There is no more tragic situation than the progressive loss of all available access sites in a patient on dialysis. We have seen gross occlusive vascular disease leading to gangrene of finger tips in a 19-year-old with advanced primary glomerulonephritis. We consider careful assessment of peripheral vessels a vital part of patient selection, and since the iliac vessels may be patent in the presence of severe distal arteriopathy, a factor in balancing choice between dialysis and transplantation. We include in our preliminary care a stern warning to other clinicians to 'keep off the veins'.

1.4 THE INFLUENCE OF SYSTEMIC DISEASE IN SELECTION

For a long period renal replacement was confined to patients without generalized systemic disorders because of shortage of facilities, and later because of a natural reluctance to be involved with further problems in a treatment already complicated enough. The commoner disorders in this group are amyloidosis, systemic lupus and diabetes. Results in the treatment of amyloidosis are encouraging in our personal experience and in that of others, even though amyloid changes may occur in a grafted kidney[9]. Results have been even more encouraging in systemic lupus.

The treatment of renal failure in diabetics has been more controversial. So often, as with a patient we are considering now, diabetic nephropathy reaches end-stage only when a patient is blind from retinopathy, with muscle weakness and with distal gangrene from peripheral neuropathy and when the access sites are virtually unavailable because of vascular occlusion. Rapid progression of retinopathy in the first year has been a major problem[10] and survival on haemodialysis relatively short[3], although results may be better with peritoneal dialysis. Transplantation seems to offer more favourable chances for rehabilitation. Overall survival figures in Europe for these diseases, taken from the EDTA Registry[3], are summarized in Table 1.1. There is no doubt that physician-effort and rehabilitation-failure are greater in diabetics than others and they are likely to rate a lower priority when dialysis places are limited.

TABLE 1.1   Survival rates of patients with diabetes, amyloidosis and lupus erythematosus in hospital dialysis

	Number	6 months	1 yr	2 yrs
Diabetes	491	83.2 ± 1	68.2 ± 3	50.0 ± 4
Amyloidosis	212	78.2 ± 3	64.4 ± 4	52.6 ± 5
Lupus erythematosus	139	84.1 ± 3	73.7 ± 5	65.4 ± 6

From the Combined Report of the European Dialysis and Transplant Association Registry 1975[3].

A word should be included about hepatitis B. In some countries this is taken relatively lightly, but in the UK strict isolation and screening of patients has virtually eliminated this problem from renal units, apart from special 'yellow' units and a few home patients. Unfortunately a new patient found to be hepatitis B positive will have great difficulty finding a place in a UK dialysis/transplant programme. Hopefully the new hepatitis vaccines may help to solve the problem.

1.5   AGE IN SELECTION

Perhaps the most controversial factor in selection is the age of the patient. During the early years of renal replacement most centres concentrated upon treating the 15–45 age group and regrettably in parts of Britain we are still nearly as restrictive. Whilst this younger group has the best survival and rehabilitation rate, several studies have now confirmed the success of dialysis in the older age groups[11] – even into the seventies. For older patients expectations should necessarily be more restricted and sensible judgement is demanded. Transplantation too is promising in the over-fifties, but survival rates to date are poorer than for younger patients or for dialysis and there is a tendency to consider dialysis as offering a better survival prospect for most older patients.

Dialysis and transplantation in children has also been an emotive issue.

There is little doubt about the success of these techniques in children although the problems of ensuring normal growth and puberty have yet to be solved. Most feel that transplantation offers better chances for full rehabilitation. Parental, if not sibling, donations are most frequently available for this group. Nephrologists once felt reservations about putting children through demanding regimens with uncertain long-term prospects, but the successes recorded for the 10-plus age group have been reassuring. These doubts still linger for very small children, with their lack of understanding, prospects of dwarfing and uncertain long-term prognosis. The techniques need to be improved.

In terms of psychological and social rehabilitation our worst prospects have been in the 13–17 age group, surprisingly. Alternation between over-dependance, distorting the whole family, and bitterness – with an often aggressive expression of the desire not to compete in a life for which they can see little long-term hope – has blighted technically successful treatment. Perhaps we have paid insufficient attention to the psychological and social needs of this group.

1.6 PSYCHOLOGICAL AND SOCIAL FACTORS

Attempts to select patients on psychological grounds have proved particularly difficult. While one tends to exclude those who are frankly psychotic, we have had considerable success in patients with a background of intermittent depressive illness. Psychiatrists often express the view, even in prospective studies, that their assessment of suitability differs little from that of the experienced clinician, although perhaps couched in more elegant terms. To some extent this reflects the natural disinclination of the psychiatrists to be cast in the role of executioner – for 'unsuitability' may equal death in uraemia. Certain personality characteristics, difficult in the management of most illnesses, are particularly troublesome in renal replacement therapy. The most worrying are over-dependance, denial – with the inevitable difficulty in collaborating with dialysis or the immunosuppressive regime of transplantation – and aggression. The patient who voices his resentment against his illness by aggression towards family and nursing staff or towards himself, is particularly difficult to manage in the close and regular contact of a renal unit. Self-aggression may take the form of fluid over-indulgence or the more dramatic form of separating shunts, cutting fistulae or discontinuing immunosuppression. Neurotic pre-morbid personalities often settle well. The remarkable stability of most individuals despite the chronic stress of a life-threatening illness is one of the most interesting and heartening aspects of dialysis and transplantation.

We have not found it easy to predict reactions to dialysis and transplantation from early response to dietary restriction – a factor some centres have stressed. Whilst one may be able to observe the aggressive, the obviously 'psychopathic' or the frankly stupid, we have had patients, most uncooperative on modified Giovanetti diets, who have flourished on dialysis and vice versa. One might anticipate better rehabilitation with a good transplant, but one lonely country lass, who coped with home dialysis well, down on the farm, and hardly ever bothered the unit, has become almost totally dependant now she has a graft with a creatinine clearance of 90 ml/min. A most valuable factor in success is a stable family background and suport from either spouse, relatives or friends. Intelligence helps (more than education) but even those of low IQ can cope.

1.7 CHOICE OF TREATMENT

Selection involves not only admission to the treatment programme, but the type of treatment to be considered. Most UK centres run an integrated home/hospital dialysis/transplant programme. The unstable, with poor support or inadequate housing, are clearly best treated at hospital or transplanted. For those who live far away home treatment has proved highly successful. We have touched on the medical indications for treatment selection between dialysis and transplantation. The interesting difference

TABLE 1.2   Home patients as a percentage of total on haemodialysis (if more than 10.0%)

	Country	1975	(1974)	(1973)	(1972)
1	United Kingdom	65.8	(64.8)	(61.6)	(58.8)
2	Ireland	36.6	(41.2)	(31.7)	(31.9)
3	Fed. Rep. of Germany	29.5	(29.0)	(27.2)	(24.2)
4	Sweden	23.1	(24.2)	(24.7)	(18.7)
5	Switzerland	21.8	(18.7)	(18.2)	(11.7)
	EUROPE	19.2	(18.8)	(18.5)	(17.6)
6	Denmark	15.4	(10.0)	(4.3)	(2.1)
7	Norway	14.1	(10.0)	(21.7)	(23.8)
8	France	12.5	(9.4)	(11.2)	(10.0)
9	Netherlands	11.4	(11.2)	(9.1)	(8.2)

in philosophy or social customs between nations is shown in Table 1.2 which reflects the percentage of dialysis patients treated at home. It is interesting to speculate whether in the UK enthusiasm for and emphasis on home dialysis has actually slowed up the development of new hospital centres, thereby contributing to our present shortfall in facilities.

The choice between home dialysis and transplantation may be difficult. Considerations of age, family support or availability of dialysis access sites may influence this choice but, despite the relative survival figures[2], most patients opt to have a transplant should one become available.

1.8 TIMING OF TREATMENT

Finally, selection should include a proper assessment of the correct timing for each phase of treatment. Where dialysis places are limited there is a risk that patients may develop severe cachexia, pericarditis, fluid overload or die before treatment is started. No hard and fast rules can be given, but the stage at which the patient is likely to lose time from work, or is becoming disabled by uraemic symptoms unresponsive to diet or is moving into negative nitrogen balance with steady loss of muscle (excluding any nephrotic phase with preservation of adequate GFR) is the time to start regular dialysis. This often corresponds to a serum creatinine greater than 1000 μmol/l, or a glomerular filtration rate below 10 to 15 ml/min. Many centres would start sooner. There is a very definite place for considering transplantation without preliminary dialysis if a suitable donor kidney becomes available. As transplantation results improve, this approach may become more commonplace.

1.9 CONCLUSIONS

For most or all of us, the unhappy early period of restricted availability of dialysis and transplantation, requiring careful selection of patients on grounds of medical and social suitability, cooperation, personality, etc., is a thing of the past. Yet in many centres, certainly in the UK, facilities remain inadequate and selection criteria still operate with regard to age and complicating medical conditions, despite the success of these treatments for a wide spectrum of age and primary illness. This shortage has the added disadvantage that treatment may be started late and patients with failing transplants may not be returned to dialysis in time. Since renal replacement therapy has a better success rate than treatment provided without question for many other fatal disorders, it is incumbent upon nephrologists to plead their cause to those responsible for selecting health care priorities. The very accurate costing of our therapies when compared with the ignorance about costing in so many other fields of medicine is an undoubted disadvantage.

ACKNOWLEDGEMENTS

I am grateful to the Editors of the Proceedings of the European Dialysis and Transplant Association for permission to reproduce Figures 1.1 and 1.2.

References

1. Quinton, W. E., Dillard, D. H., Cole, J. J. and Scribner, B. H. (1962). Eight months' experience with Silastic-Teflon bypass cannulas. *Trans. Am. Soc. Artif. Int. Organs*, 8, 236
2. Jacobs, C., Brunner, F. P., Chantler, C., Donckerwolcke, R. A., Gurland. H. J., Hathway, R. A., Selwood, N. H. and Wing, A. J. (1977). Combined report on regular dialysis and transplantation in Europe, VII, 1976. *Proc. Eur. Dial. Transpl. Assoc.*, 14, 4
3. Gurland, H. J., Brunner, F. P., Chantler, C., Jacobs, C., Schärer, K., Selwood, N. H., Spies, G. and Wing, A. J. (1976). Combined report on regular dialysis and transplantation in Europe, VI, 1975. *Proc. Eur. Dial. Transpl. Assoc.*, 13, 3
4. Cameron, J. S. and Turner, D. R. (1977). Recurrent glomerulonephritis in allografted kidneys. *Clin. Nephrol.*, 7, 47
5. Huyer, J. R., Raij, L., Vernier, R. L., Simmons, R. L., Najarian, J. S. and Michael, A. F. (1972). Recurrence of idiopathic nephrotic syndrome after renal transplantation. *Lancet*, ii, 343
6. Couser, W. G., Idelson, B. A., Stilmant, M. M., Migdal, S. D. and Davis, R. C. (1975). Successful renal transplantation in focal glomerular sclerosis: report of two cases. *Clin. Nephrol.*, 4, 62
7. Bengtsson, U. (1974). Phenacetin and renal pelvic carcinoma. *Clin. Nephrol.*, 2, 123
8. Quellhorst, E., Schuenemann, B. and Doht, B. (1977). Treatment of severe hypertension in chronic renal failure by haemofiltration. *Proc. Eur. Dial. Transpl. Assoc.*, 14, 729
9. Wilson, R. E. (1976). Transplantation in patients with unusual causes of renal failure. *Clin. Nephrol.*, 5, 51
10. Silfkin, R. F., Neff, M. S., Baez, A., Gupta, S., Mattoo, N. and Haimov, M. (1976). Maintenance dialysis in diabetic patients. *Proc. Eur. Dial. Transpl. Assoc.*, 13, 377
11. Brunner, F. P., Giesecke, B., Gurland, H. J., Jacobs, C., Parsons, F. M., Schärer, K., Seyffart, G., Spies, G. and Wing, A. J. (1975). Combined report on regular dialysis and transplantation in Europe, V, 1974. *Proc. Eur. Dial. Transpl. Assoc.*, 12, 3

DISCUSSION

R. Gabriel (London): Dr Robinson said a clearance of 5–10 ml/min. for taking people on dialysis. Did he really mean that?

Robinson: Yes, I did. I purposefully did not mention figures because I think that it is very difficult. One could certainly take higher rates, 15–20 ml/min.

Robson: What was the concentration of creatinine in the blood of your dialysis patients prior to going on to the programme?

Robinson: About 1000 μmol/l.

J. M. Bone (Liverpool): Until recently we had no hospital facilities for sustaining patients awaiting a transplant, and we had to take patients on the waiting list for transplantation without prior dialysis. This was not very successful. The transplant operation carried a 25% mortality and the waiting list itself carried a 60% mortality because patients used to die before kidneys became available. At present this is not a very good substitute for adequate supporting dialysis facilities for the transplant programme.

Robinson: I entirely agree. To get good results from transplants one must be prepared to take the patients back. We have noticed this very much within the last year or two. We have been comparing the results of patients treated by home dialysis alone with those transplanted from home dialysis. There is no doubt that the mortality rate of the transplanted group is higher and yet, nevertheless, the vast majority of patients still wanted to be considered for transplantation. Since we have been more inclined to take patients back on to a dialysis programme when the transplant has failed, and not to push immunosuppression too far, results in terms of patient survival – if not graft survival – have been much better.

One may transplant a patient before he comes on to a dialysis programme, but if good survival rates are to be achieved one must be prepared to start dialysis should the graft fail.

H. Elliott (Glasgow): Has peritoneal dialysis any value as a maintenance form of treatment, particularly in the diabetic group?

Robinson: It probably has. We have very little experience of this. We have had few patients on peritoneal dialysis. Those who have gone into it enthusiastically have claimed some very good results and there are claims that for diabetics it may be the treatment of choice. They may fare better on peritoneal dialysis than on haemodialysis, but I have no experience myself.

Has Dr Elliott any experience?

Elliott: It is very limited. Perhaps two patients.

2

The status of haemodialysis
W. R. Cattell

2.1 INTRODUCTION

Twelve years ago the potential for saving life by artificial means was the subject of great controversy[1]. In respect of kidney machines the profession was suspicious and divided; the lay public emotional and vociferous. Regular haemodialysis was being pioneered on soft money and often in the teeth of opposition from the establishment. Newspapers carried banner headlines and committees were set up to assess its acceptability. In 1965 the then Minister of Health, Kenneth Robinson, agreed that regular dialysis had passed from being a research undertaking to a proven and acceptable form of treatment which should be provided within the National Health Service. Twelve years later where have we got to? How readily available is regular dialysis treatment and how successful has it proved to be?

2.2 SUPPLY AND DEMAND

The first and perhaps crudest approach is to examine the number of patients receiving treatment at the present time. Statistics are provided by the excellent work of the EDTA Registration Committee, to whom I am indebted for the figures for the year ending 1975[2] and the provisional data for the year ending December 1976[3]. From this information we see (Table 2.1) that in December 1976 there was a total of 2409 patients receiving

TABLE 2.1   Patients receiving haemodialysis in the UK in December 1976[3]

Hospital	802
Home	1607
Total	2409
Total/mill. pop	43.0

haemodialysis treatment in Great Britain of whom 1607 or 67% were being treated in the home. Relating this to our population, a figure of 43.0 per million is obtained. I had hoped to give updated comparisons between the British performance and that in other European countries in December 1976. Unfortunately the cross-checking of this information by the EDTA Registration Committee is not yet complete and we must, therefore, be content with the 1975 data. Table 2.2 shows the rating as of December of that year. The United Kingdom comes 12th in the list, providing treatment for fewer patients than the European average. This table tells its own tale. Looking at the preliminary data for 1976 the league table is much the same.

TABLE 2.2   Comparison of haemodialysis statistics in Europe in 1975[2]

	Pop.in mill.	Hospital	Home	Total	Total/ mill.
Israel	3.4	341	14	355	104.4
Luxemburg	0.3	28	—	28	93.3
France	52.8	4067	583	4650	88.1
Switzerland	6.4	437	122	559	87.3
Fed. Rep. Germany	61.8	3565	1491	5056	81.8
Italy	55.8	3889	300	4189	75.1
Belgium	9.8	701	30	731	74.6
Netherlands	13.6	799	103	902	66.3
Denmark	5.0	247	45	292	58.4
Sweden	8.2	269	81	350	42.7
Greece	9.0	365	—	365	40.6
United Kingdom	56.0	741	1427	2168	38.7
Europe	491.4	18116	4305	22421	45.6

The position is, however, even worse than this! The data we are looking at relates to patients established on haemodialysis – some possibly for years. In assessing the adequacy of our programmes we should, however, relate supply to demand. Several studies in the United Kingdom have calculated that there are some 33 patients per million per year up to the age

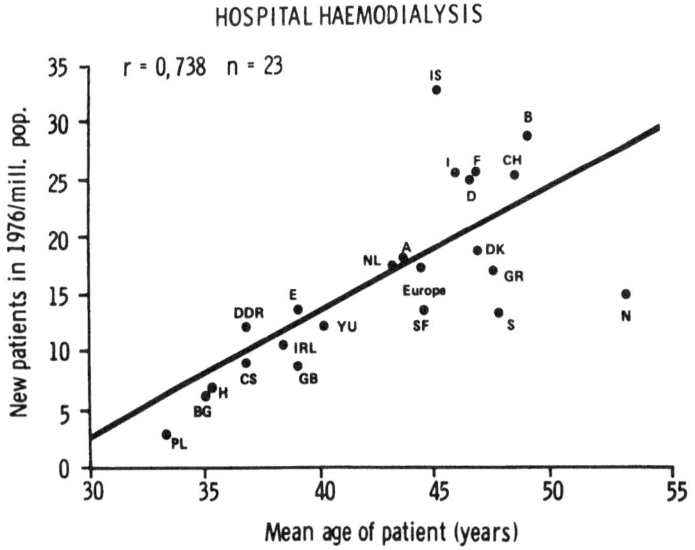

HOSPITAL HAEMODIALYSIS

Figure 2.1   Number of new patients commencing haemodialysis in 1976[3]

of 55 requiring and suitable for regular dialysis treatment. If supply is to meet demand a comparable number of patients should start regular dialysis treatment each year. Looking at the recent EDTA data, however, (Figure 2.1) we see that in Great Britain less than 10 patients per million commenced dialysis in 1976, i.e. a third of the calculated number requiring treatment. This compares with almost three times that number starting treatment in 1976 in France, Germany, Italy, Switzerland and Belgium. Interestingly, only Israel among the EDTA countries approaches the stated required level.

Another interesting point deduced from these statistics is that, with some exceptions, the fewer the patients accepted for treatment, the younger their age. This is open to several interpretations. It could be that some

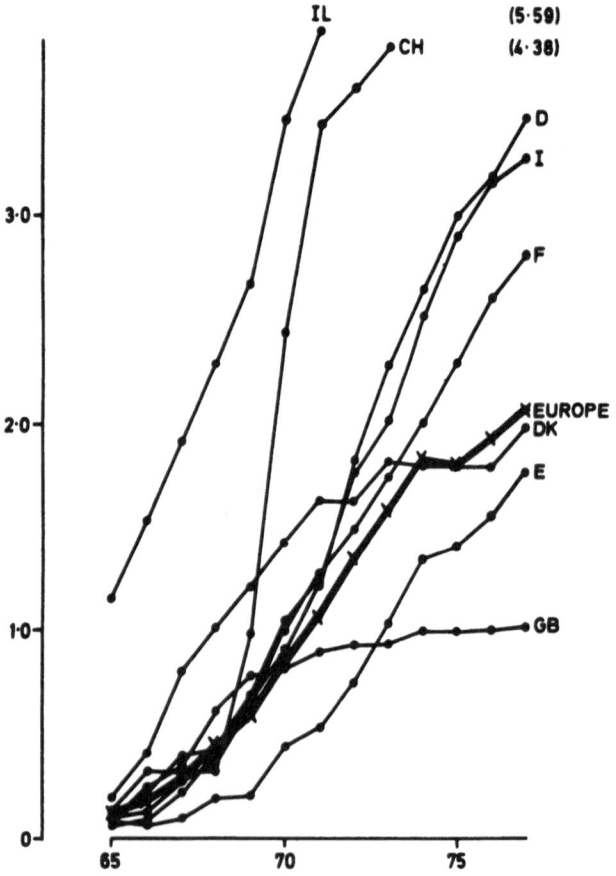

Figure 2.2   Number of centres in European countries 1965–76[3]

countries, at an early stage of development of regular dialysis facilities, elected to take older patients. Examining the countries in question this cannot apply to Holland, Ireland and United Kingdom, all of whom have been undertaking dialysis for many years. There are many other possible interpretations but the most probable is that where resources are limited, clinicians practice selection and in this age is an important factor. The more generous the facilities the greater the number of older patients that can be reasonably accepted for treatment.

This, of course, implies that we are trying to match the need. The statistics suggest we are indeed working quite hard. Thus (Figure 2.2) the United Kingdom has fewer centres per million population than most other countries, yet (Figure 2.3) we treat more patients per centre than any other European country.

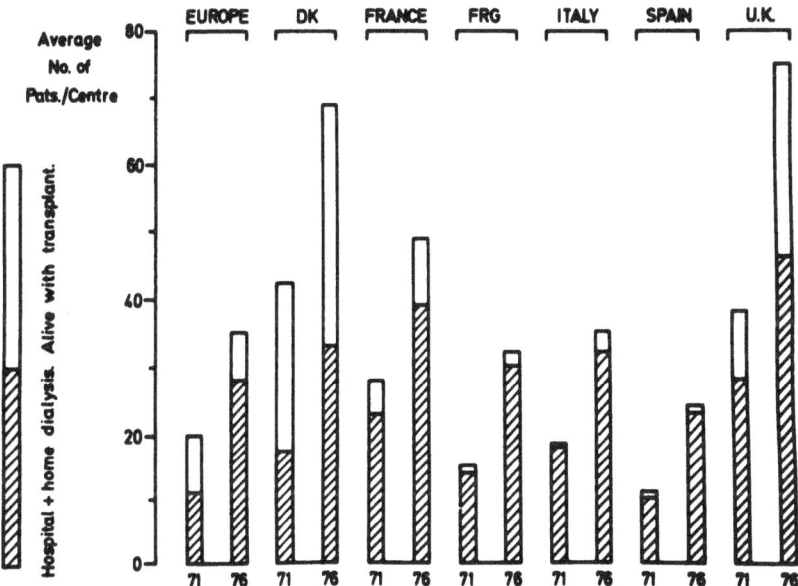

Figure 2.3   Number of patients per centre, 1971–76: all Europe and some countries[3]

The message would, therefore, seem to be that in the UK we are not in any way matching the demand for treatment despite a high workload per individual centre. As a so-called industrialized nation we should be doing better. Looking at the European data it is difficult to escape the conclusion that what we need is more centres. Thus we already have a high workload per centre and from personal experience we are all too well aware of immense demands made on staff – medical, nursing and ancilliary – to sustain this workload. To expand it further could well break the back of the system and is unlikely, rapidly, to match supply to demand.

2.3   THE QUALITY OF TREATMENT

Crude statistics on the *quantity* of dialysis provided does not, of course, necessarily reflect the *quality* of treatment. In discussing the position of haemodialysis it is thus also appropriate to ask how good is it? It is difficult to assess the quality of treatment in an otherwise life and death situation. At the risk of oversimplification I have chosen to examine it in terms of effectiveness and acceptability.

2.3.1   Effectiveness

In terms of effectiveness I have used the parameters of survival, rehabilitation, patient well-being and freedom from complications.

2.3.1.1   *Survival*

Over the past seven years the EDTA Registration Committee has carefully documented the survival statistics of patients on regular dialysis treatment in Europe. These have stayed remarkably constant over recent years with an overall 5-year survival of between 70 and 80%. Patently, when compared with other killing disease such as malignant disease or chronic bronchitis which require long-term treatment, these are excellent results. On superficial examination of the statistics, home dialysis would seem to have a better survival record than hospital dialysis but this is almost certainly qualified by selection policies and local expertise. In centres providing both there is little difference in results.

2.3.1.2   *Rehabilitation*

What, however, is the quality of this survival? One measure of this is the degree of rehabilitation as judged by the return to full-time work by those *capable and wishing* to undertake full employment. This year's analysis by the EDTA Registration Committee gives the results set out in Figure 2.4.

It can be seen that some 65% of home dialysis patients wishing to do so returned to full-time employment – essentially the same as those with successful cadaver transplants. It should, however, be pointed out that further analysis shows that, with time, patients with successful transplants over-

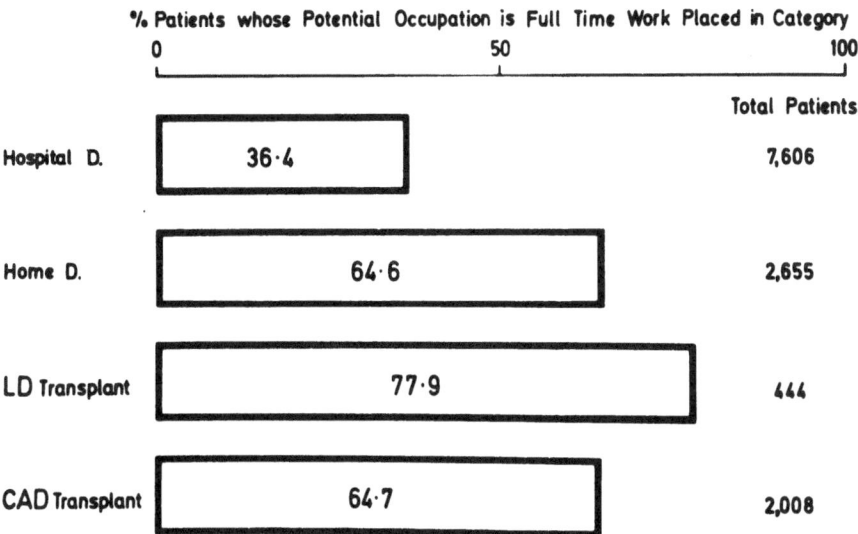

Figure 2.4   Rehabilitation of patients able and wishing to return to work[3]

take patients on home dialysis in terms of rehabilitation, reaching a 71% return to full-time work after 2 years. Hospital dialysis has a much poorer showing in terms of rehabilitation, but this almost certainly relates to selection, complications and possibly age. It is also true that many patients not rehabilitated on regular dialysis treatment, including hospital dialysis, can be returned to full-time work after successful transplantation.

2.3.1.3 *Patient well-being*

Well-being also means 'how do you feel'? We must admit that a significant proportion of patients feel less than fit. Many factors, both physical and psychological, are involved. High among these is the chronic anaemia of renal failure. Despite claims for androgen therapy or the use of cobalt, I believe that across the country as a whole we still fail to achieve really satisfactory correction of the chronic anaemia of dialysis patients and that this is one of the most important limiting factors in returning our patients to a sense of complete well-being.

2.3.1.4 *Freedom from complications*

This brings me to complications and the great success story in the UK with respect to viral hepatitis. Alone in Europe, or indeed in the world, we seem to have conquered the yellow peril. This has only been possible, however, by strict attention to preventive measures. There is a feeling abroad that we may be becoming complacent and lax. This must be guarded against. Thus it may well be less dangerous and possibly, with respect to transplantation, even advantageous to ease up on our policy of minimal transfusion, but this should only be allowed with the strictest control of screening of transfused blood for hepatitis B antigen.

What is the present situation in respect to other complications? Bone disease, dialysis dementia and hypertension will all be dealt with later. Aside from 'Newcastle bone disease' I believe that we have the increased understanding and potential to both prevent and treat bone disease and hypertension. With respect to the control of hypertension and fluid overload the selective use of ultrafiltration has been a major recent advance. Its tremendous value is already accepted in acute renal failure and in patients starting regular dialysis. Its role in the management of long-term haemodialysis is yet to be assessed, as is that of diafiltration.

What few of us have yet faced up to, however, is the prospect of ageing dialysis populations. Experience in long-established centres indicates that with advancing age of our patients and the increased incidence of vascular disease we are almost certainly going to have problems and a significant return of home patients to centre or limited care dialysis. This will be inevitable and will demand increased hospital resources.

2.3.2 Acceptability

Turning to the acceptability of regular dialysis, this may be considered under a variety of headings.

2.3.2.1 *Ease of treatment*

First and foremost, how easy is it? We have more than 10 years' experience in dialysis for chronic renal failure in the UK and should by now have refined our practice both in terms of safety and ease of operation. Have we? Critical to the performance of regular haemodialysis is satisfactory access to the circulation. This was the first important breakthrough made by Scribner and his colleagues[4] in 1960 when they introduced the Teflon shunt. Shunts have their problems and were replaced in the 1960s by the Cimino–Brescia arterio-venous fistula[5]. This in turn was an important advance but we cannot pretend that we don't have fistula problems. Indeed the ease of needling fistulae, the adequacy of blood flows obtained and fistula failure are still considerable problems. Single-needle dialysis was introduced as long ago as 1970[6] but has not received universal acceptance. Why? Partly cost and partly doubt as to its efficacy. I suspect many of us have not pursued this practice with sufficient vigour or enthusiasm. A national reappraisal of both the fistula problems and single needle dialysis would be immensely valuable in highlighting possible areas for improvement. For the present I fear that access to the circulation is still an important factor limiting the ease and efficiency of dialysis.

Regarding the hardware available, there is no doubt this has improved considerably in the past 12 years. More reliable electronic circuitry, effective deaeration, compact high performance dialysers and automated re-use equipment have all made the practice of haemodialysis *potentially* much simpler and safer. Sadly new capital equipment is expensive and many of us are still struggling with equipment bought 10 years ago with no money to replace it. More than that, modern equipment and especially disposable dialysers are associated with high running costs. With multiple reuse of dialysers costs can be reduced. With automated closed systems reusing both dialysers and lines the needs for expensive major home conversions may also be reduced. The cost effectiveness and ease of dialysis must therefore take account not only of individual units of equipment but of the whole system. However, with the possible exception of work done by Mansell and Wing[7] on the Redy system there has, as yet, been no systematic study of interrelated capital and revenue costs with modern systems. We suspect that in the United Kingdom a whole variety of different systems are in use and that dialysis costs vary considerably from centre to centre. While in no way suggesting restriction in choice of system I believe that there is an urgent need for a nationwide assessment of running costs with different systems to assess how we can best provide the easiest effective dialysis with the smallest acceptable expenditure. Individual units cannot themselves test out each different system but a multicentre analysis might well give us the answer.

This is the second time I have mentioned national multicentre studies. I think this also reflects the status of haemodialysis in the United Kingdom. Ten years ago we were all obsessed with getting our departments running and proving that we could successfully undertake regular dialysis. In those days we had the 'Dialysis Group' in this country. This met occasionally and was a forum for exchanging experience. As we got confident, the dialysis group wound up. Now, however, we could, with great benefit, pool our national experience on the various outstanding problems with great profit to our patients.

2.3.2.2   Duration of treatment

Aside from the ease with which treatment can be carried out, an important feature of acceptability is the duration of dialysis. This is a very confused area. In the very early days of regular dialysis disastrous results with poor rehabilitation and the so-called 'under-dialysis syndrome' led to the belief that it was essential to dialyse for at least 28–30 h per week. It became accepted that dialysis time was required to remove toxic compounds. There followed passionate interest in the 'middle molecule' as the offending toxin. In the past 5 years however we have seen such concepts stood on their heads. Thus we have seen a steady reduction in dialysis time with none of the dire complications predicted. Part of this may relate to more efficient dialysers with high blood flows but this is not the whole story. The importance of middle molecule in the uraemic syndrome is being seriously questioned and indeed we are really no further forward in precisely identifying what we are or should be removing by dialysis. Possibly the most important factor is control of fluid and electrolyte balance and adequate nutrition.

Whatever the theoretical implications of short-hour dialysis, in practice it seems to work and reduction in the time required for treatment has improved the acceptability of dialysis immensely. Conservative Britain is still, however, very cautious. Partly this may be because we make more extensive use of Kiil type dialysers than hollow-fibre or multiple-layer high performance dialysers. The impression gained is that we are certainly not doing less than 5 h thrice weekly or anything near the 3 h thrice weekly practised in some European centres. I suspect we are too cautious and must move with the times.

Related to short hours is of course the need to individualize dialysis. It is naive to believe that all patients, whatever their size, require or desire the same duration of treatment. It is also naive to believe that patients require the same amount of dialysis at all times. This is especially important as we reduce the hours. We must all be alert to the fact that short hours is basic treatment. If there is intercurrent infection or illness, hours must be temporarily increased. The normal kidney has reserve capacity. The artificial kidney does not.

2.3.2.3   Social convenience

Also related to the acceptability of dialysis practice is its social convenience. Assessing this is again difficult and must be related to individual circumstances. If you live in a large mansion, the butler runs your dialysis, and your social secretary plans your week. It can be organized very nicely. If you live in a two room council house with four children it is not so easy. Overall advances in the ease of treatment and reduction in hours have led to improved social acceptance. The British policy of home dialysis, dictated primarily by cost, has been successful. It is, however, too rigid. Just as duration of dialysis should be individualized so too should the site of treatment. Some patients are best suited by home dialysis while others would be happier with limited care centre dialysis. This must be equated with the financial resources available but I believe we should now be moving to more flexibility into how and where we treat our patients both for social as well as for economic reasons.

2.3.2.4 Dietary freedom

Finally, we cannot consider the acceptability of regular dialysis without consideration of dietary freedom. A principal function of the normal kidney is to get rid of waste material from our diet. Kidney failure demands restriction in our diet. How well does dialysis restore the freedom to eat? I think there can be no doubt that over the past 12 years we have all moved to more sensible and liberal diets for our patients. Aside from restrictions in water, sodium and potassium most patients should now be free to eat a pretty normal diet. Certainly the expensive high calorie diets formerly recommended are unnecessary in the well treated subject. In part this relates to better management of chronic renal failure prior to dialysis but mainly it relates to confidence in our dialysis capability.

2.4 CONCLUSION

In conclusion how would I summarize the status of haemodialysis in the UK? I think it reflects our national character and economic climate. It may be summarized as being responsible, reasonably industrious, decidedly conservative, definitely under-financed but successful against the odds.

ACKNOWLEDGEMENTS

I am grateful to the Editors of the *Proceedings of the European Dialysis and Transplant Association* for permission to reproduce Tables 2.1 and 2.2, and Figures 2.1, 2.2, 2.3 and 3.4.

References

1. Fox, R. C. and Swazey, J. P. (1974). *The Courage to Fail. A Social View of Organ Transplants and Dialysis*. (London: University of Chicago Press Ltd.)
2. Gurland, H. J., Brunner, F. P., Chantler, C., Jacobs, C., Schärer, K., Selwood, N. H., Spiers, G. and Wing, A. J. (1976). Combined Report on Regular Dialysis and Transplantation in Europe, VI, 1975. *Proc. Eur. Dial. Transpl. Assoc.*, **13**, 3
3. Jacobs, C., Brunner, F. P., Chantler, C., Donckerwolcke, R. A., Gurland, H. J., Hathway, R. A., Selwood, N. H. and Wing, A. J. (1977). Combined Report on Regular Dialysis and Transplantation in Europe, VII, 1976. *Proc. Eur. Dial. Transpl. Assoc.*, **14**, 3
4. Quinton, W., Dillard, D. and Scribner, B. H. (1960). Cannulation of blood vessels for prolonged hemodialysis. *Trans. Am. Soc. Artific. Inter. Org.*, **6**, 104
5. Brescia, M. J., Cimino, J. E., Appel, K. and Hurwich, B. J. (1966). Chronic hemodialysis using venipuncture and a surgically created arteriovenous fistula. *N. Engl. J. Med.*, **275**, 1089
6. Panter, H. R., Kopp, K. F., Gutch, C. F. and van Dura, D. (1972). Single needle dialysis. *J. Extracorp. Technol.*, **4**, 41
7. Mansell, M. A. and Wing, A. J. (1976). Long term experience of home dialysis with sorbent regeneration of dialysate. *Proc. Eur. Dial. Transp. Assoc.*, **13**, 275

DISCUSSION

A. C. Kennedy (Glasgow): I would agree with both the previous speakers in their analysis of why we have fallen down the league table in respect of the number of patients treated. Over-dependence on home dialysis may well be a factor and we do not have enough centres. It is not that we do not work hard enough.

There is, I believe, a further factor. To a certain extent we operate under career restraints. Those who are in charge of dialysis units were themselves trained as physicians and nephrologists, and we lack the facility to have dialysis centres run by career dialysers who would only do dialysis. It is that kind of a possibility that has allowed, say, Italy to take off in an upward direction and to increase markedly the number of patients on dialysis. I am not advocating that we should do this. I doubt if we could under our career structure and training system, but it is a factor.

Robson: I was delighted to hear Dr Cattell identify a role for the community physician. They certainly need a role and it would be nice to be able to offer them some suggestions.

B. H. B. Robinson (Birmingham): The figure showing the development of new centres is really quite striking – the change in the slope for the UK, which occurred when the Ministry of Health stopped financing directly and left everything to the regions. There was a slowdown then, and there has been total stasis since the reorganization of the Health Service.

It is not just the money. There is a blanket of bureaucracy at the moment.

Cattell: I accept Professor Kennedy's first point. If he means a career dialysis doctor, then there are one or two in Britain who are first class. I am a great believer in the barefoot doctor and we have reached the level of sophistication in dialysis where we could probably run several dialysis centres without the doctor involvement that we have at the moment, and I should like to see this happen.

There has been a restriction on the number of new centres since reorganization. It is difficult to interpret. The original committees set up by the DHSS to plan home dialysis set certain targets. There were to be so many centres per unit of population and home dialysis would serve a hundred-plus patients. Possibly the nephrologists have been slightly 'hoist with their own petard' in that they thought that each centre could handle far more patients than it does.

Robson: But I am sure it was the way to begin. There was no other way. The issue is whether it is the way to go on.

3

Current status of renal transplantation
D. N. H. Hamilton and J. D. Briggs

3.1   INTRODUCTION

In an ideal transplanter's world any patient on regular dialysis would prefer an offer of a living donor transplant or a well-matched healthy cadaver kidney. In the real world organizational and immunological problems prevent this ideal, and clinical compromise is essential. Even renal physicians, who are unhappy about renal transplantation, are forced by economic and organizational problems to accept transplantation in order to increase the number of patients treated because of limited dialysis capacity. There is also unanimous pressure from the patients themselves to obtain a transplant.

Thus the current status of transplantation is not the result of an overall plan, but is a shifting balance produced by two shortages – of dialysis facilities on the one hand and of donor kidneys on the other.

In discussing the status of transplantation one is thus aware of being controlled by events rather than being in control. The supply of donor kidneys, the results of transplantation and two major areas for improvement of the results will be described.

3.2   LIVING DONORS

A kidney transplanted from a relative is still the best therapy for chronic renal failure, not because of immediate function, nor entirely because of good HLA matching, but because of the success in (co-incidentally) matching non-HLA factors. Taking the figures from the European experience[1], kidney survival at one year is best with a 'full house' sibling transplant (72.5%) but less successful with only one haplotype match or with a parent to child graft (66.2%) or vice versa. Each type of living donor gives concern to the transplant surgeon for the consequences to the donor. Parents may be frail or have vascular disease; siblings may be wage earners or mothers of young children, and the willingness of informed consent from younger donors may be in doubt. It is perhaps for these reasons that in the UK the percentage of living donors is only 12% and transplant units have avoided an aggressive hunt for living donors in a family.

3.3   CADAVERIC DONORS

3.3.1   Supply

The National Organ Matching Scheme works well for distribution and matching of donor kidneys. The supply of kidneys is less than the demand,

and in 1976 the numbers of donors in the UK dropped for the first time and the number of transplants done annually seems stuck at about 300. The rate-limiting step in this supply is not the general public's attitude (all surveys show a general willingness to donate), but a disinclination of the doctors looking after the prospective donor to consider kidney donation. Transplant surgeons themselves cannot be absolved from responsibility for some of these sensitivities and perhaps private discussion and re-assurance may succeed where public remonstration has failed.

Not only are there concerns about the number of kidneys available but also about the quality.

3.3.2 Quality

While the shortage of supply of cadaveric kidneys certainly occasionally forces surgeons to use unsuitable kidneys (e.g. those with vascular or parenchymal damage or anomalies), the idea that 'dead' kidneys are being used (i.e. kidneys with severe irreversible ischaemic damage) is less soundly based. Seventeen per cent or so of cadaveric kidneys in the UK never work[2], and this figure is rising. However these kidneys may not have been killed by ischaemia. They may instead have rejected during the period of acute tubular necrosis and the available evidence, such as the good function of the partner of these 'dead' kidneys, supports this view[3]. Further investigation of this problem is important since, if 'dead' kidneys do exist, it is necessary to improve methods of collection and to use more 'heart-beating' brain-dead donors. It would also be necessary to use tests of kidney viability and to decide among the conflicting claims for these tests[4,5] (such as ATP levels, K/Na ratios, [^{125}I]iodohippuran). On the other hand, if kidneys are being rejected more frequently in the period of acute tubular necrosis, then the investigation must shift to possible changes in the immunological status of the recipient.

3.4 TRANSPLANTATION ROUTINE

The usual procedure for obtaining cadaveric kidneys, tissue typing and transplantation have been standard for some years and have been reviewed elsewhere[6]. Indeed the practice of transplantation has changed little since 1970 and many of the improvements suggested have failed to win a routine place in practice. Dr T. E. Starzl, a pioneer in kidney transplantation, recently observed in a reflective moment that the 'failure of radically new methods to be developed in the last 10 years has relegated progress to the shuffling of details'[7].

3.4.1 Selection and preparation of patients

Dialysis patients going forward for transplantation should be under 50 and reasonably fit. Excluded are those with systemic disease likely to shorten life (malignancy or severe vascular disease) or recur in the transplanted kidney (polyarteritis or oxalosis). Patients with peptic ulcers require prophylactic surgery (though some dispute this) but all agree that chronically infected or polycystic kidneys should be removed prior to transplantation and that the same procedure should be carried out in hypertensive patients. Doubts have been raised whether home dialysis patients, who have excellent survival, should be transplanted but as the majority live in hope of a transplant, it is hard to actively exclude them from this possibility. Priority for transplantation can be given to patients who have problems on dialysis (such as repeated thrombosis of access devices) though successful transplantation fails to reverse dialysis dementia. Though it is tempting to transplant patients in renal failure before any dialysis is required, the results are poor.

As for tissue typing, most units in the UK accept that tissue typing is of value to transplantation and a two-match kidney is the minimum accepted or offered.

3.4.2 Kidney preservation

In spite of considerable research efforts expended on kidney preservation, both in variants in the type of fluid used to flush the kidney and machines to maintain viability of the kidney, the majority of renal units find a simple flush with an intracellular type solution (e.g. Perfudex) is sufficient, though recently the European Cooperative Scheme have recommended Collins solution. Few units use perfusion machines as the original claims of improved kidney function and ability to be able to discriminate damaged kidneys as a result of using such machines have met a sceptical response. While it is true that the use of the preservation machine can allow transplant surgery to be carried out at leisure during office hours, most units still find it suitable to transplant within 12 hours of donation. Perfusion machines also require trained supervision, though the latest Gambro machine has many simplifications.

There are many variables involved in transplantation, making the effects of various perfusion fluids or machine preservation difficult to assess.

3.5 IMMUNOSUPPRESSION

The original, empirically derived, combination of steroids and azathioprine has been the routine therapy for 20 years. Experience with cyclophosphamide as an alternative has been disappointing and it is not now recommended[7]. There have been enthusiastic reports on the immunosuppressive properties of unsaturated fatty acids and carragenan, but full reports are awaited. Though anti-lymphocyte globulin (ALG) is a potent immunosuppressive agent in experimental animals its value in human renal transplantation has been controversial with only some centres reporting success. The method of preparation, the dosage and timing may be crucial. The problem of establishing that any ALG batch is indeed immunosuppressive in human patients is formidable, though if it gives depression of lymphocyte function or prolongation of monkey allografts, then the ALG may be judged to be effective.

3.6 TREATMENT OF REJECTION

Increased steroid dosage is always employed but local radiation to the kidney has been shown to be valueless in the management of rejection[8]. Much effort has been expended to devise tests which anticipate rejection, but though the value of some in the early detection of rejection has been established the work load required in any centre to test the whole group of recently transplanted patients each day is formidable. There also remains a suspicion that early detection of rejection may not change the outcome of a rejection episode. Direct evidence on this point would be useful.

3.7 ROLE OF TISSUE TYPING

Cooperative kidney sharing schemes like the National Organ Matching Service (NOMS) and Eurotransplant have, as their *raison d'être*, the assumption that successful matching improves the results of transplantation. The results, though, are still controversial, and large series in America and the collected data for Europe (Figure 3.1) show little or no benefit of tissue typing. Paradoxically the results from smaller cooperative groups or from individual centres (who often form part of the bigger series) show a marked benefit of tissue typing (Figure 3.2). Thus the literature on the role of tissue typing in first cadaveric transplants is confusing, but the explanation may lie in the obfuscation produced by pooling data from many centres and the variation introduced in other factors influencing the outcome. It may therefore be that the results from individual centres represent the truth of the matter.

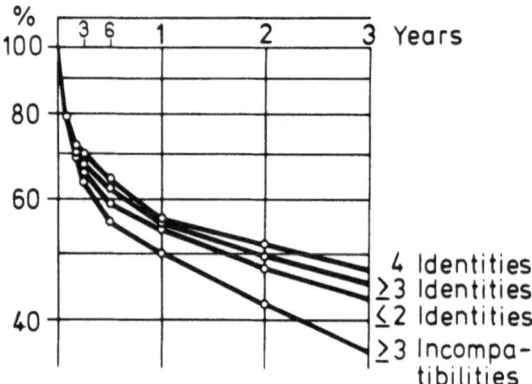

Figure 3.1   Effect of tissue typing on first cadaver kidney transplant results in collected figures from European Dialysis and Transplant Association 1975[1]

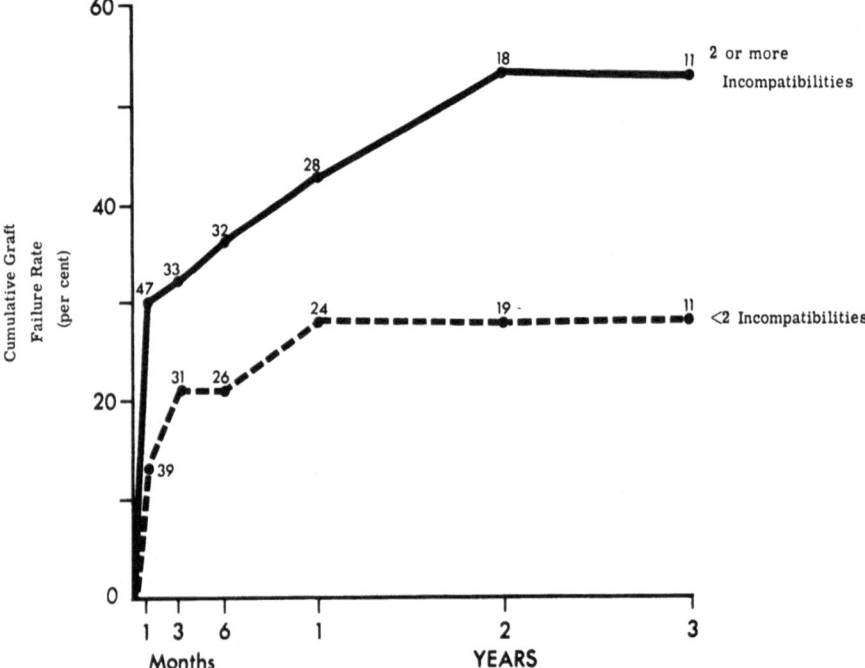

Figure 3.2   Effect of tissue typing on first cadaver transplant results in Glasgow (unpublished). In both this and the EDTA series two or more incompatibilities are compared with less than two

One well established finding from all studies is that in second cadaveric transplants tissue typing is a major determining factor, and as good a match as possible is desirable for these second transplants.

3.8   RESULTS BY YEAR OF TRANSPLANTATION

Though continuous improvement in many of the factors influencing trans-plantation has been made, this has not been reflected in the results. Indeed there has been a suspicion that some additional factor has been changing to hold back progress. In our unit we are concerned that kidney transplants are being rejected more vigorously than before. Though the results of large cooperative groups tend to obscure such changes, nevertheless the figures from the Kidney Transplant Registry in the USA also show a slight decline in survival rate. Both these figures are shown in Table 3.1. The trend in Glasgow is rather depressing but analysis shows that factors such as tech-nical failure, poorer tissue typing or alterations in policy for recipient selection cannot be blamed. An increased immunological attack on the allografted kidney seems likely, and we have looked at two possible ex-planations, namely the effects of blood transfusion and the role of endo-genous cell-mediated immunity.

TABLE 3.1   Percentage kidney survival at one year, by year of operation, of first kidney allografts in Glasgow and from the USA Kidney Transplant Register[9]

	USA	Glasgow
1969	53.7 ± 1.7	75
1971	53.0 ± 1.2	60
1973	49.5 ± 1.1	46
1975	NA	44

These two new factors give hope for progress and the hints came not from laboratory, but from clinical observations. The first was the effect of prior blood transfusion on the transplant results and the second from in-vestigations of the endogenous cell-mediated immunity (CMI) on patients receiving regular dialysis treatment.

3.8.1   Effect of blood transfusion

It was an early finding that blood transfusion could prolong allograft survival in dogs[10] and rabbits[11]. Dosseter[12] had made a similar claim for human allografts. However, it was not until Terasaki[13] called attention to

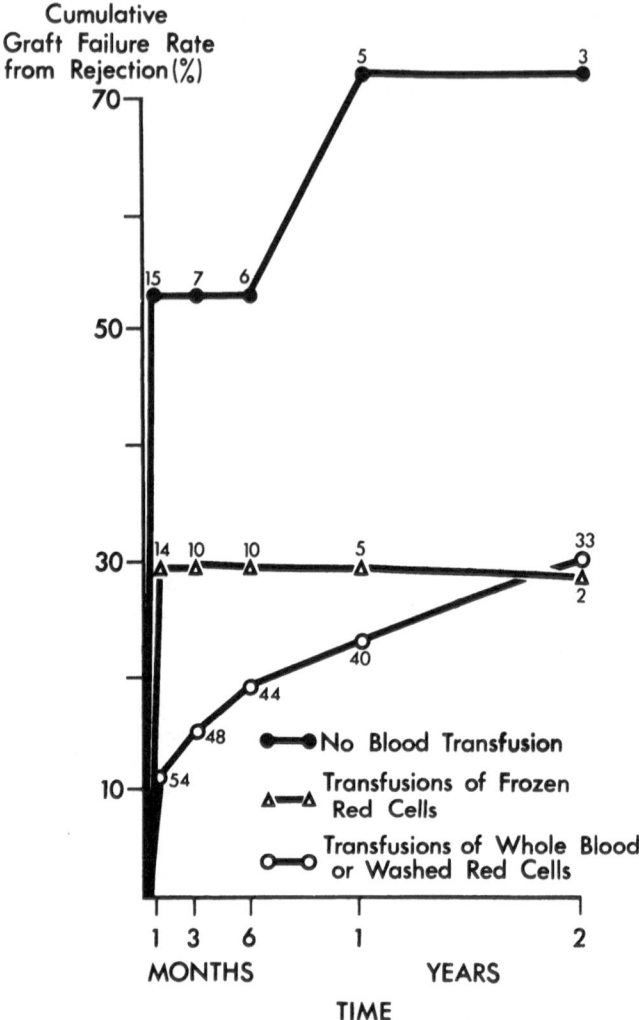

Figure 3.3   Effect of previous blood transfusion (whole or leukocyte poor) on the results of cadaveric transplantation in Glasgow (unpublished)

better kidney transplant results in transfused RDT patients that the matter was taken seriously. This finding has been confirmed in a number of studies from individual centres (Figure 3.3), though the pooled European data showed no benefit of prior blood tranfusion.

These findings do make some immunological sense since a unit of whole blood contains leukocytes bearing HLA antigens which can and do raise cytotoxic antibodies in normal and to a lesser extent in RDT patients. To explain *prolongation* of an allograft it is postulated that in some patients transfusion produces enhancing antibodies or tolerance (possibly 'low zone' in type). The suggestion however that blood transfusion *causes* prolongation of graft survival is subject to the following criticisms:

(1) Blood transfusions are not given randomly to RDT patients but for good reasons (e.g. elective surgery, gastro-intestinal bleeding or because of anaemia due to previous bilateral nephrectomy). Hence the transfused and non-transfused groups are not similar and may thus have different results after kidney transplantation.

(2) The data shows that even one small transfusion[14] is related to a better result, which would be difficult, though not impossible, to explain immunologically.

3.8.2 Immune depression and transplant results

The marked depression of CMI in RDT patients was an early finding[15] and possibly explains the unexpectedly good results in the early days of transplantation. However the outcome of kidney transplantation in indi-

TABLE 3.2 Table showing 6 month survival of first cadaver allografts according to DNCB skin reactivity prior to transplantation. Results from Johns Hopkins[16] and Glasgow (unpublished). Initial sensitization was with 2000 μg of DNCB and testing was with 200 μg

	Hopkins	Glasgow
DNCB negative	85% ($\hat{N}=45$)	84%
DNCB positive	56% ($\hat{N}=10$)	33%

vidual patients in relation to their CMI levels has not been analysed until recently (Table 3.2). Using skin testing with dinitrochlorobenzene (DNCB) as a test of cell-mediated immunity, these two studies show that RDT patients with no reaction to DNCB had a 6 months kidney allograft survival of about 80% while those with any degree of response had only a 30% kidney survival. These studies therefore shift attention away from the donated kidney and tissue typing to the host factors in allograft survival. It also shows that the CMI of RDT patients may vary and emphasizes that little is known of the biochemical or other changes in RDT patients which depress CMI though some experimental studies suggest the suppressor cells are responsible[17].

These studies also suggest that some patients may paradoxically be too fit and hence unsuitable for transplantation.

These findings on CMI levels in RDT patients and the effects of blood transfusion may offer an explanation of any recent worsening of the results of transplantation, since it may be that CMI levels in RDT patients have been rising in recent years, or that the policy of reducing whole blood transfusion during RDT has prejudiced the chance of kidney survival. Both factors do not exclude the other as an explanation and blood transfusion into anergic RDT patients may produce markedly different immunological changes compared with normal human patients.

3.9   REHABILITATION

The assessment of the results of transplantation by mortality and morbidity gives only part of the answer to the value of transplantation.

The results of transplantation are variable. Some patients have an excellent clinical result with a near normal quality of life, but some despite an excellent functioning kidney have a serious chronic disability such as repeated affliction with bone disease. Some patients, who have rejected a kidney, return to dialysis as if nothing had happened but there are those whose health and spirits are broken by the loss of the kidney and the therapies necessary to try to save it. Any attempt to assess the contribution made by transplantation in the management of patients with chronic renal failure must weigh up all clinical factors and also attempt to measure the 'quality' of life. So far assessment of results has been primitive and mainly confined to simple assessment of working capacity. As expected, of the patients covered by the EDTA Survey[1], 85% of the living-donor transplant patients were at full-time work and 76% of the cadaver donor patients were also working full-time; the corresponding figures for home and hospital dialysis were 73% and 37%. A more systematic evaluation of the 'quality' of life would be of help in attempting to assess objectively the contribution of transplantation. A successful kidney transplant is a therapeutic triumph, restoring physical and mental vigour, restoring sexual potency and function and liberating patients from the constraints of their dialysis life. Tables of graft and patient survival do not tell the whole story.

ACKNOWLEDGEMENTS

We are indebted to the Editors of the *Proceedings of the European Dialysis and Transplant Association* for permission to reproduce Figure 3.1.

References

1. Parsons, F. M., Brunner, F. P., Burk, H. C., Graser, W., Gurland, H. J., Harlen, H., Schärer, K. and Spies, G. W. (1975). Statistical Report. *Proc. Eur. Dial. Transpl. Assoc.*, 11, 3
2. British Transplantation Society Report (1975). *Br. Med. J.*, 1, 251
3. Hamilton, D. N. H. and Briggs, J. D. (1975). Kidneys for transplantation. *Lancet*, ii, 461
4. Williams, G., Peet, T. N. D. and Hamshere, R. J. (1976). Assessment of a test of renal viability. *Br. Med. J.*, ii, 75
5. Sells, R. A., Mcloughlin, R. A. and Tyrrell, I. (1974). Renal cortical cation composition as an index of human kidney graft viability. *Br. J. Surg.*, 61, 326
6. Briggs, J. D. and Hamilton, D. N. H. (1976). Transplantation in Scotland. *Hlth. Bull.*, 34, 190
7. Starzl, T. E., Weil, R. and Putnam, C. W. (1977). Modern trends in kidney transplantation. *Transpl. Proc.*, 9, 1
8. Godfrey, A. M. and Salaman, J. R. (1976). Radiotherapy in treatment of acute rejection of human renal allografts. *Lancet*, i, 938
9. 13th Report of Human Renal Transplant Registry (1977). *Transpl. Proc.*, 9, 9
10. Halasz, N. A. (1963). Enhancement of skin homografts in dogs. *J. Surg. Res.*, 3, 503
11. Billingham, R. E. and Sparrow, E. M. (1955). The effects of the prior intravenous injections of dissociated epidermal cells and blood on the survival of skin homografts in rabbits. *J. Embryol. Exp. Morph.*, 3, 265
12. Dosseter, J. B., Mackinnon, K. R., Gault, M. H. and Maclean, L.D. (1967). Cadaver kidney transplants. *Transplantation*, 5, 844
13. Opelz, G. and Terasaki, P. I. (1974). Poor kidney-transplant survival in recipients with frozen-blood transfusions or no transfusions. *Lancet*, ii, 696
14. Van Es, A. A., Marquet, R. L., Van Rood, J. J., Kalff, M. W. and Balner, H. Blood transfusions induce prolonged kidney allograft survival in Rhesus monkeys. *Lancet*, i, 506
15. Dammin, J. (1956). Prolongation of skin graft survival in uremia. *Ann. N.Y. Acad. Sci.*, 64, 967
16. Rolley, R. T., Sterioff, S., Parks, L. C. and Williams, G. M. (1977). Delayed cutaneous hypersensitivity and human renal allotransplantation. *Transpl. Proc.*, 9, 81
17. Johnston, M. F. M. and Slavin, R. G. (1976). Mechanism of inhibition of adoptive transfer of tuberulin sensitivity in acute uremia. *J. Lab. Clin. Med.*, 87, 457

DISCUSSION

F. M. Parsons (Leeds): Are the effects of blood transfusion an artefact? May I expand on that?

A patient who has not been transfused has not been challenged with foreign protein. If a patient is transfused there is an immunological challenge. Are we perhaps picking up that challenge in the form of circulating antibodies and discarding such patients from transplantation? In other words, are we selecting in such a way that the so-called 'weak responders' are transplanted? Has this anything to do with it?

Hamilton: I do not know whether originally we distinguished between responders and non-responders. But now, looking at the whole group of transfused patients, including those who may have had some cytotoxic antibodies, if they are transplanted after careful cross-matching they do better as well.

The responder/non-responder idea seems to have faded a little. What might be interesting is to try to relate the response to blood transfusion with the skin testing results. The anergic patients are unlikely to respond with cytotoxic antibody, but they may make another kind of antibody. The whole problem keeps coming back to the immunological state of the dialysis patients and their response to blood transfusion.

Robson: Mr Hamilton's results are quite remarkable, and very like six or seven others in the literature. I have heard it asked whether it is ethical to conduct controlled trials of the effect of blood transfusion. There have now been six reports, all pointing in the same direction.

Hamilton: I do think that it is ethical. This is the last chance to do a controlled trial − just at this point. There are so many artefacts possible, especially the selection of patients, that we must do it.

Wallace (Glasgow): We should remember that the main reason for introducing frozen red cells into the dialysis and transplant units was to reduce the risk of hepatitis. We have had a warning (today) that the hepatitis may be lurking just around the corner. We sometimes place too much emphasis on hepatitis B and we forget that there are other infective agents, such as cytomegalovirus, and that there are good reasons for continuing to use frozen blood cells to reduce the dangers of infection. I doubt whether we have enough evidence to discontinue their use. I am in favour of multi-centre trials.

Hamilton: I take the point. CMV virus is not thought to be the major cause of morbidity considering the number of transplant patients that are infected with it, although I am not minimizing it.

Robson: A controlled trial cannot be carried out with frozen red blood cells because they do not have the immunological effect.

Hamilton: It is the white cells, of course, that may give the effect.

R. Gabriel (London): On the frozen blood story, could I ask whether it is the patient's own blood that is being taken and put under nitrogen, or anybody's blood, and with or without white cell separation.

Hamilton: It is certainly not the patient's own blood. It is donated blood and the white cells are separated physically.

Wallace: The best method of producing so-called leukocyte-poor and platelet-poor blood is to use red cells recovered from frozen banks. One must never use the term 'leukocyte-free' or 'platelet-free'. It is leukocyte-poor and platelet-poor so that there is still the possibility of immunization to HLA antigens or other antigens which may be more important than HLA within the nature of the histopathological complex.

Robson: It is surely true that where frozen red cells are used for transfusion there is apparently no immunological advantage over those patients given no blood. There have been several reports pointing in that direction. If a controlled trial is to take place it has to be with blood, not frozen.

It is rather ironic that as time has passed and we have reduced the reasons for not putting people on dialysis, e.g. systemic disease, or multiple myeloma, we are forcing ourselves into a much more difficult moral position. Ten years ago it was a great relief to find a patient with chronic renal failure who could not be transplanted because of a myeloma, or a little bit of lupus, or some other reason for not doing it. Now that this is being removed, the ethical dilemma becomes much worse in relation to the shortage.

Parsons: I have a further comment to Dr Cattell.

Having been in the European Registry, I have some inside information. One of the reasons why the UK is falling behind its neighbours is – regrettably – the gross national product. If the number of patients per million of population is plotted against the gross national product of any country, then the UK is slap on the line. In other words, we are living up to our income, as it were. If we want to get across the need for more money for patient care – may I be political? we must get it across to the miners that it is no good their asking for £135 per week. We need more money in the Health Service. How are we to do that?

Robson: I am sure that is so, but it seems extraordinary. The UK is among the industrial nations on superficial social assessments, and yet dialysis-wise it ranks with Greece, Portugal, and the unindustrialized nations.

Parsons: Which is correct on a comparison with the gross national product. I do not believe that we in the UK appreciate that we are so poor!

W. R. Cattell (London): This is from an analysis which correlates GNP per head of population. What Parsons says is correct. A slope showing many of the so-called industrialized nations on it has the UK way along the line. However, it is not fair to say that any of the so-called industrialized nations are allocating out of their GNP an appropriate amount for replacement therapy. I have only seen the slide once, but I believe that Israel is way off the line, spending far more per million population than it ought to do along the line made up by the other poorer nations. Is that correct?

Parsons: No, it is not. Israel is a special case. It so happens that during the past 2 years expansion of the number of dialysis centres has been phenom enal, hence the new intake has been phenomenal as well. A fall-off can be expected in future years.

Robson: And that is a sad state of affairs.

SECTION TWO

Economics and Limited Care
Chairman:
Sally Taber

SECTION TWO

CONNECTING SOLUTIONS

4

The economics of treating chronic renal failure
D. M. Parkin

4.1   INTRODUCTION

Effective treatment for chronic renal failure became a reality in the early sixties with the development of intermittent haemodialysis and renal transplantation. By 1975, it was apparent that there were considerable international differences in the proportion of potential patients who received treatment. It seems likely then that there are constraints which limit the development of treatment programmes, one of which is certainly the level of finance available. This paper will consider some of the economic aspects of treating chronic renal failure.

4.2   SIZE OF THE PROBLEM

The potential number of patients requiring treatment must be estimated from epidemiological surveys of renal failure. There have been several in the UK[1-3], the most recent of which in Scotland suggested that about 96 patients per million total population under the age of 65 die annually from chronic renal failure. Of this number 52 per million have no intercurrent disease which would tend to contraindicate treatment. Under the age of 55 corresponding numbers are 63 per million total, and 38 per million 'suitable' for treatment.

In the UK in 1975 the number of new patients commencing treatment was about 14.5 per million population, which is a much lower proportion than in any other EEC country (except Ireland)[4]. Figure 4.1 shows the number of patients actually receiving treatment (prevalence) in the years 1972 to 1975, and, with the current annual mortality rate of 11%, the numbers who will be receiving treatment in each of the next 5 years with differing assumptions of 'intake'. The lower line represents 14.5 new patients per million population, the central line the numbers expected if the population of patients commencing treatment continues to increase at the rate experienced since 1972, and the upper line the number on treatment if intake is increased to 38 per million per year (a level already exceeded in North America, Japan and Israel).

Kerr in 1967[5] was the first to examine the economic implications of offering treatment to this number of new patients. He assumed 2300 new patients under 55 per year, and a 10% annual mortality on dialysis. With fairly modest estimates of the costs of running a hospital dialysis unit he came to the conclusion that annual expenditure would rise to £17$\frac{1}{2}$ million after only five years. Changes in survival on therapy, and the development of home dialysis and transplantation as alternatives to hospital care, render the conclusions of the analysis less valid today. Nevertheless it elegantly

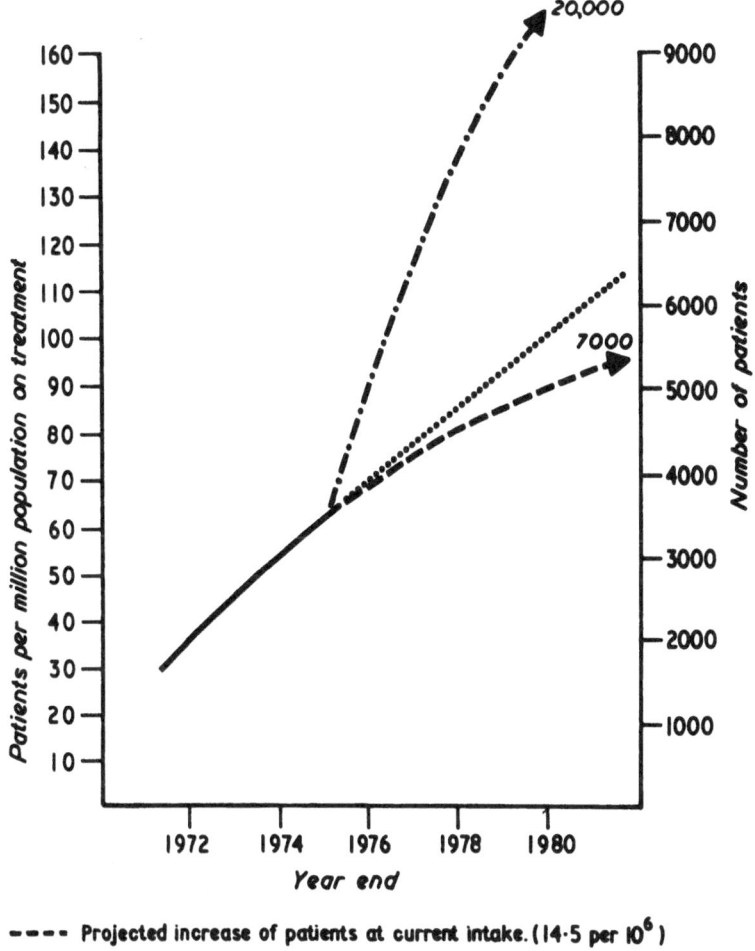

Figure 4.1   Actual and projected numbers treated (dialysis and transplant) UK, final equilibrium at 7000 and 20 000 respectively

demonstrated the principle that the development of effective therapy for a chronic disorder leads to a rapid increase in prevalent cases requiring treatment, until new cases (represented by the incidence rate) are balanced by deaths, or transfers to other forms of treatment (transplants). A complex model illustrating the full development of this principle has been developed by Farrow *et al.*[6].

4.3 COST OF TREATMENT

A study of the economics of managing renal failure requires that some costs are put upon different modalities of treatment. Chronic intermittent haemodialysis was developed as a hospital technique and there have been attempts to estimate the costs of treating patients in hospital. There are great difficulties in doing so, not least because of problems of apportioning capital costs (machines, buildings) on a 'per patient per year' basis. For what they are worth figures from different centres are shown in Table 4.1, together with estimates of running costs (excluding capital equipment) for the UK.

TABLE 4.1   Costs of hospital dialysis

Author	Year of estimate	Place	Annual cost (1975 £ equivalent)	
A: Annual total cost per patient				
Klarman et al.[7]	1968	USA	$14 000	(11 000)
Pearson et al.[8]	1972	USA	$14–25 000	(9–16 500)
Douglas[9]	1972	USA	$20–30 000	(13–20 000)
Schippers and Kalff[10]	1973	Netherlands	$26 000	(16 000)
Stewart et al.[11]	1973	Australia	$A 7 400	(6 000)
Buxton and West[12]	1972	UK	£5 600	(8 800)
B: UK Annual revenue costs only				
Kerr[5]	1967		£1 470	($3 175)
DHSS[13]	1970		£2 000	($3 710)
Farrow et al.[6]	1971		£2 500	($4 200)
Buxton and West[12]	1972		£3 900	($6 100)

Treatment at home is undoubtedly less expensive than treatment in hospital, in addition to having other advantages. Costs are easier to estimate than those of hospital care, since a price for equipment and home adaptation is relatively easy to obtain. The only problem is in apportioning part of the cost of the 'back up' hospital unit to each home dialysis patient, since all patients require initial training in a hospital unit, and some will require subsequent readmission for complications. Some estimates of capital costs and maintenance are shown in Table 4.2. Approximate present costs in Leeds are £4000 for equipment (machine, monitor, dialyser) £1500 for home adaptations and an annual running cost of £2250 per patient per year.

Obtaining the cost of a renal transplant is even more of a problem, and since there are no units which are devoted entirely to this activity, separat-

TABLE 4.2 Costs of home dialysis

Author	Year of estimate	Place	Capital cost*†	Maintenance*
Klarman et al.[7]	1968	USA	—	$5 000 (4 000)
Pearson et al.[8]	1972	USA	—	$5 600 (3 700)
Rae et al.[14]	1972	Canada	$8 750 (5 700)	$5 854 (3 800)
Douglas[9]	1973	USA	—	$4–6 000 (2 500–4 000)
Stewart et al.[11]	1973	Australia	$A6 000 (4 800)	$A2 600 (2 100)
Hull[15]	1975	USA	—	$15 600 (7 600)
Kerr[5]	1967	UK	£3 500 (7 600)	£1 150 (2 500)
DHSS[13]	1970	UK	—	£1 500 (2 800)
Farrow et al.[6]	1971	UK	—	£1 000 (1 700)
Robinson[16]	1971	UK	£2 450 (3 600)	£1 300 (1 900)
Buxton and West[12]	1972	UK	£3 800 (5 900)	£2 700 (4 200)
Ogg[17]	1973	UK	£3 000 (4 400)	£2 000 (2 900)

* 1975 sterling equivalent in brackets.
† Includes equipment, home adaptation and 'training'.

TABLE 4.3 Costs of a renal transplant

Author	Year of estimate	Place	Cost of operation	Cost of follow-up
Klarman et al.[7]	1968	USA	$13 000 (10 000)	—
Kountz[18]	1969	USA	$10 000 (7 500)	—
Douglas[9]	1972	USA	$13–16 000 (8 500–10 500)	—
Schippers and Kalff[10]	1973	Netherlands	$18 000 (11 300)	$3 200 (2 000)
Stewart et al.[11]	1973	Australia	$A8 900 (7 100)	$A800 (700)

Figures in brackets= approx. 1975 sterling equivalent.

ing the cost of a transplant patient from hospital running costs is almost impossible. No one in the UK has ever published a guess. Some figures from other countries are produced in Table 4.3. The actual values by themselves mean little, but comparing them with dialysis costs it can be seen that a transplant operation probably costs less than dialysis for one year in hospital.

4.4 IS IT WORTH IT?

The foregoing discussion has indicated the enormous potential expenditure on treatment for chronic renal failure. The implicit question therefore arises about the proportion of our health service finance that should be spent on such treatment. In a wholly logical world a health service planner would be faced with a series of independent programmes and could choose between them, one element guiding his choice being the return on the money he invests. This is the basis of the cost-benefit approach to medical care. Some weighing of benefit against cost goes on in many fields of medical decision making, and although many doctors reject such a notion as somehow unethical, I believe it is better to be as explicit as possible about the basis of our decisions, rather than relying upon subjective value-judgements.

There have been two attempts at relating costs to benefits in regard to treatment of chronic renal failure. The first of these by Longmore and Rehahn (1975)[19] involved some curious assumptions and calculations. These authors markedly underestimated costs of treatment, assumed that all patients treated return to full-time employment, made no allowance for mortality of treated patients, and did not 'discount' the value of a patient's future earning to their present value[20,21]. A more satisfactory analysis was performed by Buxton and West (1975)[12]. I will not discuss their methods in detail, but merely present here some of their assumptions and conclusions. They examined a theoretical cohort of 1000 patients commencing therapy by dialysis, either in hospital, or at home, and utilized mortality rates and rehabilitation rates provided by EDTA for 1972. The costs of treatment at 1972 prices were estimated for hospital as £5600 per year per patient, and for a home dialysis patient £3390 per annum with an initial cost of £1300. Benefit to society was assessed in terms of average earnings for males and females respectively, in the proportion of patients able to work. The use of those earnings which would have been lost as a result of premature death as a means of assessing benefit to society has been challenged[22], but although unsatisfactory in many ways, this is a perfectly reasonable way of estimating what are termed 'indirect benefits' of a programme[23]. Buxton

and West do however fail to consider the 'direct benefits' of treating
patients – that is the immediate, tangible savings to the health service. In
this case these savings would be the excess cost of caring for 1000 patients
dying of renal failure at present as compared with their terminal care as
they die, on treatment, over the ensuing 20 years under consideration.

At the time of their analysis the conclusions reached were that the 1972
value of benefit of treating 1000 patients was about £3.6 million for hospital dialysis, and £6.3 million for home dialysis (the latter figure is higher
because of better survival/rehabilitation on home dialysis, this of course
reflecting selection criteria for home dialysis training). The 1972 cost of
maintaining the same cohort on treatment for 20 years was £23 million for
hospital dialysis, and £20 million for home dialysis. This yields cost-benefit
ratios of 6.4 : 1 for hospital care, and 3.2 : 1 for home care.

As already discussed Buxton and West exclude consideration of 'direct'
benefits. Percentage survival and rehabilitation have also increased since
1972 (see EDTA 1975 data[4]), and improvements in hardware and techniques have probably resulted in a relative lowering of costs. These factors
will all lower the cost-benefit ratio. In addition, as the authors admit, no
mention is made of renal transplantation as a possible 'cheap' option in
treatment. Nevertheless, I believe that the conclusion that there is no
positive economic return from the treatment of renal failure is valid.

Society is in fact tacitly agreeing to pay for 'intangible benefits'[23], that
is the avoidance of pain, discomfort, grief and the premature loss of human
life. These are exceedingly hard to measure in financial terms, and though
economists may attempt it, the medical profession is on the whole averse
to doing so. I believe it is this that makes cost-benefit so difficult to apply
in the health field.

4.5 VALUE FOR MONEY

Assuming that treating patients with renal failure is not a financially rewarding exercise, but that society is prepared to do so for the sake of the
intangible benefits, the next question is how to get 'the best value for
money'. Here we are concerned with cost-effectiveness of treatments and
procedures: what is the most economical way of achieving a given outcome? This type of analysis is much easier than cost-benefit, since benefits
do not need to be costed in financial terms. In its simplest form we can
examine the cost of one life-year saved by different forms of treatment.
Pioneering work by Klarman et al. (1968)[7] took this approach, in comparing haemodialysis with transplantation. The authors in addition allowed
for the putatively superior quality of life after transplantation, valuing such

TABLE 4.4   Present value of expenditure and life-years gained per member of cohort embarking on transplantation and in-centre and home dialysis

Modality	Present value of expenditure	Life-years gained	Cost per life-year
Dialysis			
Hospital	$104 000	9	$11 600
Home	$38 000	9	$4 200
50–50 programme	$71 000	9	$7 900
Transplantation			
Unadjusted	$44 500	17	$2 600
Adjusted for quality	$44 500	20.5	$2 200

Note: Cost of transplantation incorporates $24 500 for dialysis based on a 50–50 distribution of patients between hospital and home.

(After Klarman *et al.* 1968[7])

a life-year 25% more highly than one on haemodialysis. The results are demonstrated in Table 4.4. This work is now almost 10 years old, and it is perhaps not surprising that many of the assumptions it contains require revision, in particular the projected results for transplantation appear optimistic both in terms of graft and patient survival, and the 'life-years gained' figure is certainly too high. Nevertheless, others have reached the same conclusions about the relative expense of dialysis and transplantation, for example DHEW in the USA estimates a life-year costs $6300 on dialysis, and $3500 after transplantation (cited in Douglas 1973[9]).

4.6   CONCLUSIONS FROM COST DATA

The most economical method of treating renal failure appears then to be by transplantation. This has a high (and difficult to estimate) initial cost of operation and post-operative care, as well as an initial outlay on dialysis whilst awaiting a suitable organ. After operation, costs are relatively small (drugs and out-patient attendances), but mortality is quite high, 40% at 3 years; in addition the majority of grafts will fail in the same period (Figure 4.2)[4], so that many of the surviving patients will require a return to dialysis care. Even allowing for this, however, cost per life-year is lowest for this form of treatment, as well as offering the most satisfactory quality of life.

All workers agree that home dialysis is cheaper per patient-year than hospital dialysis. There are however considerable differences in the relative costs depending upon what is counted under each heading, and the proportion of a hospital unit costs which are allotted to 'necessary support' for a home dialysis programme. Survival in hospital (65% at 3 years) is poorer than that at home (81% at 3 years), although this of course largely reflects selection of patients; survival rates on home dialysis can only be calculated

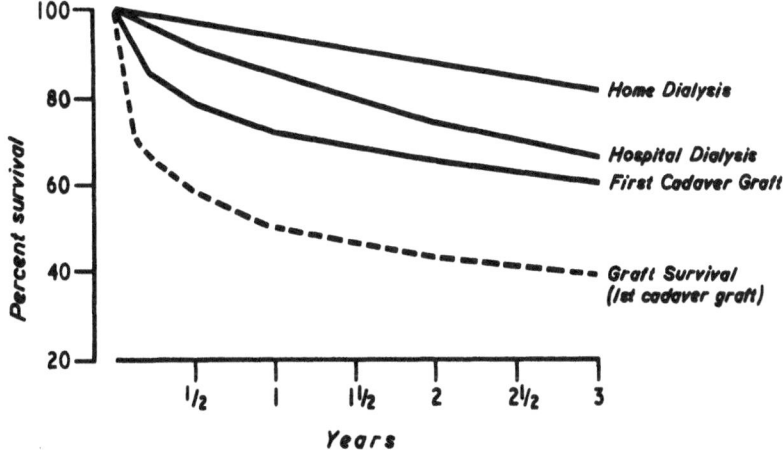

Figure 4.2   Cumulative patient survival. Europe 1975
(After Gurland et al.[4])

after the patients have already been treated in hospital, cases who are 'poor risks' will either die in this period, or continue in hospital care (Figure 4.2). Likewise the degree of rehabilitation achieved by patients is better for home dialysis than hospital care, and is almost as good as that of trans-

TABLE 4.5   Rehabilitation and mode of treatment
Europe 1975[4]

Mode of treatment	Total patients	Working full-time (%)	Working part-time (%)	Able to work, not doing so (%)	Unable to work (%)
Hospital dialysis	15 489	33.8	24.8	20.9	20.4
Home dialysis	3 827	64.1	15.7	14.0	6.2
Transplant	4 083	67.7	12.0	13.2	7.1

plant patients (Table 4.5). One of the many reasons for the better rehabilitation of patients treated by home dialysis is probably because the timing of treatment can be individually adjusted to be outside normal working hours.

4.7 THE BALANCE OF TREATMENT METHODS

The discussion so far has looked at the economic implications of different forms of treatment as if these were independent. Of course this is not so, and in practice it is necessary to adopt a mixture of different methods. Hospital dialysis is an expensive procedure, and by itself could not support a treatment programme of any size without an enormous increase in facilities. In practice patients are removed from the hospital dialysis pool by transplantation, by transfer to home dialysis, or to some form of limited care. Farrow et al.[6] constructed a model of a treatment programme for renal failure involving dialysis (hospital and home) and transplantation, and were able to study the theoretical effects of varying the proportions receiving different treatments.

Although their costing data is rather inadequate, they used their model to look at the economic implications of different treatment programmes[24]. Reliance on dialysis (home and hospital) alone produces an expensive programme, with good survival figures. The addition of transplantation leads to poorer overall survival, but there are advantages in terms of lower costs, and increased numbers of patients who can be treated with fixed facilities.

4.8 INTERNATIONAL COMPARISONS

It is instructive to look at the treatment of renal failure in different countries, and how the different methods of financing treatment has led to differing balances in the use of resources. The UK is now (1975) 17th in an international league table comparing patients on treatment per million population, behind all the EEC countries, Scandinavia, the USA and Japan[4]. It is impossible to say exactly what this means in terms of total national resources devoted to treating renal failure without knowledge of incidence rates, but there is a suggestion of a rough correlation between a nation's wealth and the amount spent on renal disease (Figure 4.3).

The UK had 53 centres offering dialysis in 1975, a ratio of 0.9 per million population, much lower than any other Western nation. This policy of restricting the number of dialysis places in hospital has undoubtedly been responsible for the UK having the largest proportion of dialysis patients on home treatment (65.8% of all dialysis patients in 1975). The more abundant hospital facilities elsewhere mean that a smaller proportion of patients have been trained for home dialysis, despite the undoubted economic benefits of doing so. An additional effect of restricting hospital facilities has been to increase the proportion of renal failure patients treated

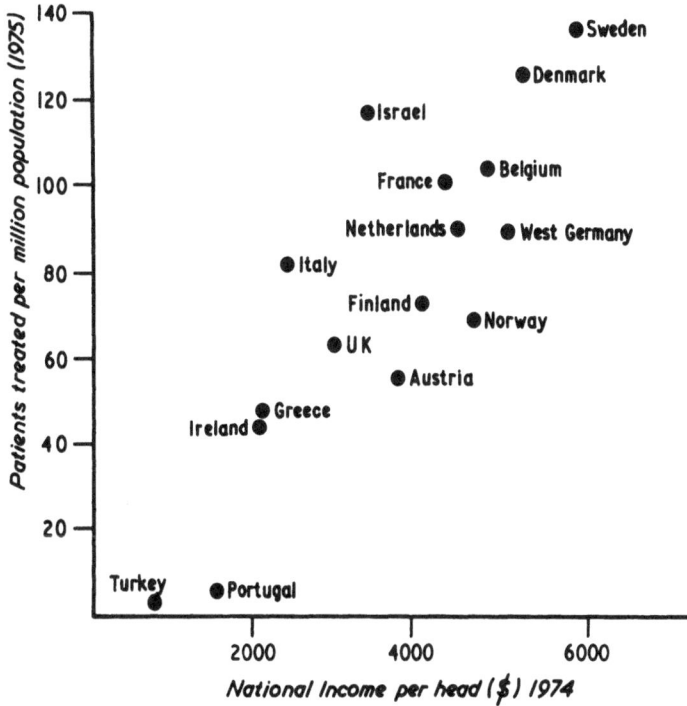

Figure 4.3   Treatment for renal failure in relation to national income

by transplantation. The UK is the only European country to demonstrate this cost-effective trend between 1971 and 1976[25].

The influence of finance on treatment patterns can be seen from recent US experience (Figure 4.4). In 1973 the Federal Government began to finance dialysis and transplantation via Medicare. Prior to this the financial advantages of home dialysis had been evident in the increasing proportion of patients using this modality. Since 1973 a patient attempting home dialysis is faced with expenses which are not covered under Medicare, but which would be covered if he was an out-patient at a facility[26]. The result has been a fall in the proportion of home dialysers and an increasing proportion using 'limited care' facilities. The economics of 'limited care' are considered later, but according to Jenkins et al. [27], the result of this change is an increased cost of treatment, the burden of which falls upon federal tax-payers.

The economic advantages of transplantation as a form of therapy have already been described; the limitations upon this form of treatment seem to be the supply of suitable donors' organs. In Australia early formulations of

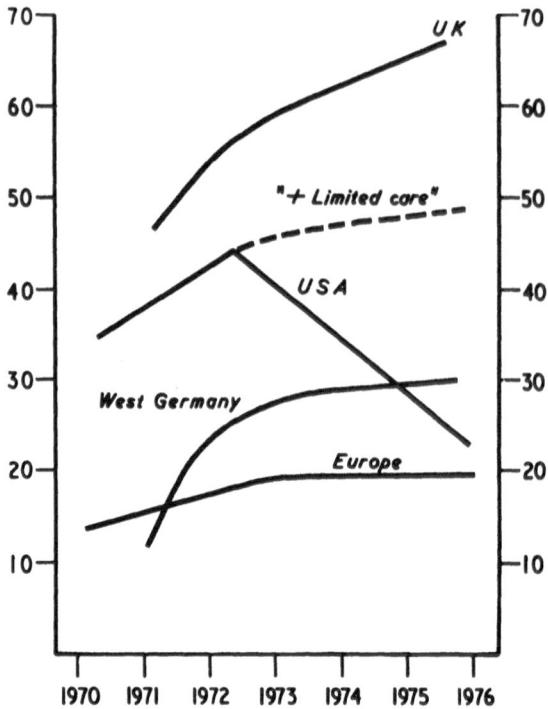

Figure 4.4   Proportion of patients on dialysis treated at home (1975)
(After Gurland *et al.*[4])

policy for treating renal failure sought to use a combination of hospital
dialysis with early transplantation[28], both of which were government
financed, in contrast to home dialysis, which was not. Stewart *et al.*[11] have
shown the medical and economic implications of this 'early transplant'
policy as opposed to home dialysis with elective transplantation. Interestingly this produces similar conclusions to those reached by Farrow *et al.*[24]
with their theoretical model, i.e. hospital plus early transplant leads to
poorer survival, but the cost per surviving patient is considerably less than
the home dialysis/elective transplant model.

4.9   THE ECONOMICS OF LIMITED CARE

Limited-care dialysis involves the patient attending a 'facility' as an out-
patient, and in the USA these facilities have developed as 'Satellite Centers'
outwith hospitals[29,30]. Reduced expenses on buildings and staffing means
that such centres are considerably cheaper to operate than hospital units.

They have an advantage over self-dialysis at home in that capital costs, including equipment, are shared by more than one patient and that death or successful transplantation do not mean relocation. However, staffing and travel costs generally make it more expensive than home treatment in the long term. Bilinsky *et al.*[31] estimate costs per dialysis as $128 hospital, $65–69 in satellites and $46 at home. The proportion of patients dialysing in limited care facilities has shown a remarkable increase in the USA in recent years. As already discussed this has probably developed as a relatively cheap alternative to hospital care in the face of the financial disincentive to home dialysis.

4.10 CONCLUSIONS

From an economic viewpoint, renal transplantation is the most effective method of treating chronic renal failure. However, the number of transplants per year in the UK, just over 6000, accounts for only $\frac{1}{3}$ to $\frac{1}{4}$ of the renal failure patients who require treatment. The number of transplants performed is not increasing[32]. The results of transplantation will probably improve with more effective tissue matching and better immunosuppressive therapy, but currently it is scarcity of donor organs that limits the number of operations. Six years ago Crosby *et al.*[33], in a retrospective survey of hospital deaths, found a potentially adequate supply of donor kidneys. Efforts to eliminate this constraint on treatment would undoubtedly be worthwhile.

Other than transplantation the only practical long-term solution to treatment lies in dialysis, either at home or in limited care satellites. There is little experience of limited care in the UK, but there is no reason to suppose that they would be more cost-effective than home dialysis for long-term treatment, since lower capital costs per patient would be rapidly overtaken by greater running costs. Limited care units may well be a useful alternative to hospitals for certain patients who are unable to manage themselves at home and also possibly an economical proposition in the short-term management of patients awaiting a transplant.

Cost-benefit study tends to suggest that there is no overall financial gain to society from treating patients with renal failure. This in no way implies that we should not seek to do so, it merely adds a piece of information which assists in the attempt to achieve some rationality in the use of health care resources. It is for health professionals to persuade society to allot as many resources as possible for health care, so that maximum help can be given to sufferers from renal failure, amongst other groups.

ACKNOWLEDGEMENTS

My thanks are due to Dr A. M. Davison, Renal Unit, St. James's Hospital, Leeds, and Dr J. L. Anderton, Medical Renal Clinic, Western General Hospital, Edinburgh, for their helpful comments and criticisms of the draft of this paper. I am indebted to the Editors of the *Proceedings of the European Dialysis and Transplant Association* for permission to reproduce Figures 4.2 and 4.4.

References

1. Branch, R. A., Clark, G. W., Cochrane, A. L., Jones, J. H. and Scarborough, H. (1971). Incidence of uraemia and requirements for maintenance haemodialysis. *Br. Med. J.*, 1, 249
2. McGeown, M. G. (1972). Chronic renal failure in Northern Ireland, 1968–1970. A prospective survey. *Lancet*, ii, 307
3. Pendreigh, D. M., Heasman, M. A., Howitt, L. F., Kennedy, A. C., Macdougall, A. I., Macleod, M., Robson, J. S. and Stewart, W. K. (1972). Survey of chronic renal failure in Scotland. *Lancet*, i, 304
4. Gurland, H. J., Brunner, F. P., Chantler, C., Jacobs, C., Schärer, K., Selwood, N. H., Spies, G. and Wing, A. J. (1976). Combined Report on Regular Dialysis and Transplantation in Europe, VI, 1975. *Transpl. Assoc.*, 13, 3
5. Kerr, D. N. S. (1967). Regular haemodialysis. *Proc. R. Soc. med.*, 60, 1195
6. Farrow, S. C., Fisher, D. J. H. and Johnson, D. B. (1971). Statistical approach to planning an integrated haemodialysis/transplantation programme. *Br. Med. J.*, 2, 671
7. Klarman, H. E., Francis, J. O. and Rosenthal, G. D. (1968). Cost effectiveness analysis applied to the treatment of chronic renal disease. *Med. Care*, 6, 48
8. Pearson, D. A., Stranova, T. J. and Thompson, J. D. (1976). Patient and program costs associated with chronic hemodialysis care. *Inquiry*, 13, 23
9. Douglas, R. A. (1973). The costs of kidney transplantation and hemodialysis. *Transpl. Proc.*, 5, 1043
10. Schippers, H. M. A. and Kalff, M. W. (1976). Cost comparison hemodialysis and renal transplantation. *Tissue Antigens*, 7, 86
11. Stewart, J. H., Topp, N. D., Martin, S., Schawrowas, E., Flaus, Y., Sheil, A. G. R. and Mahony, J. F. (1973). The costs of domiciliary maintenance haemodialysis: a comparison with alternative renal replacemet regimens. *Med. J. Aust.*, 1, 156
12. Buxton, M. J. and West, R. R. (1975). Cost-benefit analysis of long term haemodialysis for chronic renal failure. *Br. Med. J.*, 2, 376
13. Editorial (1970). Demand for machines and organs. *Nature (London)*, 225, 1183
14. Rae, A., Craig, P. and Miles, G. (1972). Home dialysis; its costs and problems. *Can. Med. Assoc. J.*, 106, 1305
15. Hull, A. R. (1976). 1976 concepts of hemodialysis. *Arch. Intern. Med.*, 136, 365

16. Robinson, B. H. B. (1971). Intermittent haemodialysis in the home. *Br. Med. Bull.*, **27**, 173

17. Ogg, C. (1973). Priorities in medicine: society should be better informed. *Br. Med. J.*, **4**, 648

18. Kountz, S. L. (1969). Cited by Pearson *et al.* (reference 8)

19. Longmore, D. B. and Rehahn, M. (1975). The cumulative cost of death. *Lancet*, i, 1023

20. Buxton, M. J. and West, R. R. (1975). The cost of death (letter). *Lancet*, ii, 38

21. Glass, N. (1975). The cumulative cost of death (letter). *Lancet*, i, 1341

22. Roberts, J. A. (1975). Cost-benefit analysis of long-term haemodialysis for chronic renal failure (letter). *Br. Med. J.*, **3**, 230

23. Klarman, H. E. (1974). Application of cost-benefit analysis to health systems technology. *J. Occup. Med.*, **16**, 172

24. Farrow, S. C., Fisher, D. J. and Johnson, D. B. (1972). Dialysis and transplantation: the national picture over the next five years. *Br. Med. J.*, **3**, 686

25. Jacobs, C., Brunner, F. P., Chantler, C., Donckerwolche, R. A., Gurland, H. J., Hathway, R. A., Selwood, N. H. and Wing, A. J. (1977). Combined Report on regular dialysis and transplantation in Europe, VII, 1976. *Proc. Eur. Dial. Transp. Assoc.*, **14**, 3

26. Levine, C. (1976). Home dialysis and the Medicare gap. *Hastings Centre Report*, 6, 5

27. Jenkins, P. G., Gutmann, F. D. and Rieselbach, R. E. (1976). Self-hemodialysis: the optimal mode of dialytic therapy. *Arch. Intern. Med.*, **136**, 357

28. National Health and Medical Research Council (1968). Report of the ad hoc committee on rationalisation of facilities for organ transplantation and renal dialysis. *Med. J. Aust.*, 2, 1200

29. Johnson, W. J., Hathaway, D. S., Anderson, C. F. and Carlson, R. A. (1970). Hemodialysis: comparison of treatment in the medical center, community hospital and home. *Arch. Intern. Med.*, **125**, 462

30. Neff, M. S., Baez, A., Slifkin, R. and Schupak, E. (1973). Out-patient dialysis. *Arch. Intern. Med.*, **131**, 717

31. Bilinsky, R. T., Morris, A. J. and Klein, H. R. (1971). Satellite dialysis: an economic approach to the delivery of hemodialysis care. *J. Am. Med. Assoc.*, **218**, 1809

32. Tovey, G. H. (1976). Annual Report 1975–76 of the National Organ Matching Service of the UK.

33. Crosby, D. L., West R. R. and Davies, H. (1971). Availability of cadaveric kidneys for transplantation. *Br. Med. J.*, **4**, 401

DISCUSSION

W. R. Cattell (London): I find it very interesting that Dr Parkin has tried to tackle the question of costs. May I have clarification? When he says it costs so much to provide a transplant, is that the cost of a successful transplant, and what about the costs of the patient with a failed transplant who has to go back on dialysis? Are those costs added to the cost of the successful transplant?

Parkin: The figures I gave included the failures. If there was a transplant unit doing nothing else we could work out the number of life-years we succeed in getting by doing the operation and divide that into the money-costs. Patients whose transplants fail and who need to continue on dialysis have to be taken into account.

Cattell: So that if they fail and go back on dialysis, the money that is spent on that is added to the cost-benefit for the successes.

Parkin: Yes.

J. S. Robson (Edinburgh): The cost-benefit approach is fascinating. Sir Douglas Black has done some work on trying to assess the shape of the National Health Service in terms of life-years saved or lost by various diseases.

However, take mental deficiency, which is an enormous burden on the Health Service. I would not like to say how much it costs, but it can be expressed as 5% of the cost of the Health Service. There are no, or virtually no, life-years lost. On Dr Parkin's analysis, these patients are alive, they have to be equated with the average national income, yet they do not work. The cost-benefit to the nation of the enormous expense of keeping mental defectives alive is a higher ratio, a worse ratio, than dialysis where the patients die and cost nothing after they are dead.

I am rather challenging the validity of relating the benefit in terms of the average working input, or we must begin to compare it with different disabled groups in society.

66

Parkin: I have no wish to try to defend cost-benefit analysis in general. It is by no means the answer to everything. To try to assess the benefit to society in financial terms of a programme to treat chronic renal failure is an incredibly difficult thing to do. I happened to pick on one paper – the only one that has ever attempted to do it – and I then used the method to assess the indirect benefits by calculating the income, proportion of gross national product, or whatever that would be lost if patients were not treated. It is not a very satisfactory way of doing things, but it is incredibly difficult to think of any other way of doing it.

The point about mental deficiency is that there is no particular saving. It might be argued that in a totally cost-benefit orientated medical field, the *only* benefits are the direct financial benefits, and that therefore patients with mental deficiency should not be treated.

I did stress that there are other benefits. I called them intangible benefits. They are the social costs; the costs of death, disability, pain, grief, etc. One can try, if one likes, to put a price on those in pounds sterling, as some planners of highway systems do in comparing road and rail systems, but in general I do not see the doctors doing it.

J. S. Cameron (London): Dr Cattell has raised an important point. What happens next is that shortage of dialysis places makes transplantation appear cheaper than it really is, and this situation is probably no longer true. Since policy is determined by the sort of calculations that we have to do right now, it is important to look at the implications of this. What has probably happened in the past is that because of a shortage of dialysis places, people were not put back on dialysis after graft failure and therefore died. Death – we have already agreed – is cheap. Secondly, the transplanters and their physician colleagues pushed too hard on treatment to save failing grafts and patients died of all the horrible complications with which we are only too familiar, whereas adequate dialysis provision would allow these patients to be treated, and would allow them to return to dialysis. The cost of the failed graft does not appear in most of the analyses that are done and, until recently, the sort of mortality rate Dr Parkin showed in the graph was usual. I believe that the Australians first showed that the mortality of the patient, even when 50% of cadaver grafts were failing in the average population treated, could be pushed to less than 10% – into single figures over 5 years following the graft, even though one, two, or even three grafts were done during that time. The implications for this on the costs of transplantation and the number of dialysis places needed, given that our mortality is now down to single figures, are enormous, which reinforces further earlier statements about the need for more dialysis places and more dialysis units to support the transplant pro-grammes.

Boulton-Jones (Glasgow): Can I return to Dr Parkin's interesting slide showing the correlation between numbers treated per million against the national income. The correlation shown was most reassuring to adminis-trators because it means that we are being zealous in apportioning the funds. However, he has also said that there is a high percentage of trans-plantation and a high percentage of home dialysis patients; both of them cheaper forms of treatment. That means that we should be well above the line on the graph if we are allotting the same amount of money.

Parkin: So that the proportion of our GNP spent on dialysis and on renal disease is probably less than it should be. That is probably right.

C. P. Swainson (Edinburgh): Dr Parkin has shown very nicely how the kind of analysis he has described can help us, and can help doctors in general, to decide between different modes of treatment of the same illness. But how does he, as a health planner, begin to approach the problem of deciding the allocation of resources between similar forms of chronic illness? For example, take nephrology's main rival, heart disease.

Parkin: That is why I tentatively suggested using cost-benefit, because that is the only objective way of doing it, illogical as it is. There is no other objective way of doing it. Otherwise it is purely subjective.

We do take the financial considerations into account. Cost-benefit can be rejected as crude for looking at life-years saved and the benefits in terms of how much someone would earn. But other criteria, such as the age of patients, or whether they are diabetic, or for example the 92-year-old patient with a stroke, have to be considered in cost benefit. We do it intuitively, whether we like it or not.

Miss S. Taber: Should we not be looking at the available kidneys? Dr Parkin has said that these are limited. Perhaps we should be putting more money into improving the supply of cadaver kidneys. In the US they have a system using a transplant coordinator, run by a business organiza-tion, and they have available the numbers of kidneys that they want. More of our finances in the UK should be put to trying to improve the supply of cadaver kidneys.

Parkin: I should have thought that that was a logical conclusion. I am no expert in renal disease, but having spent some time reading through the statistics that seems to be the most obvious – apart from increasing the number of centres. I have said that there is only one centre per million, but we do very well on that. That is not to say that we do not need more. Apart from that, we should be sorting out the supply of cadaver kidneys. It should be relatively simple.

Cameron: We have no need to go to the US for this information. We should be looking harder – as Dr Cattell did in the survey which he did for the Renal Association – at the variations in service provided both in terms of dialysis and in terms of transplantation throughout the different regions of Great Britain and Northern Ireland. These variations are very large.

One of the questions which the health planners might answer is how much of the variation resides with the different structure of medical care in those areas and how much is the direct result of financial deprivation. This is capable of analysis. Some regions, including our own South-East Metropolitan Region, are already treating 38 patients per million of population per year. If we can do this because we have more cash than other regions, then there are implications for planning.

Parkin: A comparison of those areas that are doing well or are doing badly in terms of dialysis within the UK shows that they correspond quite well to the analysis of whether they are plus or minus 50% over the amount of funding. There is no doubt about that.

5

The practicalities of limited care

The need to reconsider forms of treatment for patients on long-term haemodialysis

Helen Rosenthal

5.1   INTRODUCTION

Ever since regular haemodialysis for chronic renal failure became an
accepted form of treatment rather than sheer adventurism, the debate
around the relative merits of home dialysis, hospital dialysis, limited care
and transplantation has flourished around the world. According to the pre-
occupations and prejudices of each renal unit, the superiority of one form
of treatment over another is demonstrated by the degree of patient rehabilitation, or the expressed preferences of the patient, by cost-benefit analyses
or patient survival statistics. It is salutary to view this debate in the wider
setting under which health care is delivered in a particular country. Differing health care systems subject to different forces and pressures can play
determining roles in making available particular forms of treatment. If
those determining forces and pressures continue to prevail, our need to
justify the form of treatment which we offer may blind us to the changing
needs of that most important person – the patient. Nowhere can this be
seen so dramatically as in high-cost, high-technology, highly specialized
treatments like chronic haemodialysis.

The UK has consistently led the field in home dialysis. While the
European average of patients on home dialysis as a percentage of all
patients on regular dialysis was 19.2% in 1975, the figure was 66% for the
UK. Over the preceding 5 years, the UK regularly had the highest percentage of home dialysis patients. By contrast, in the USA, there was a
rapid decrease in home dialysis over the 3 years 1972–75, from 42% to
24%. This was accompanied by a simultaneous increase in the number of
patients using limited-care facilities. This more than compensated numeri-
cally for the drop in numbers of home dialysis patients[1].

Why should there have been a sustained prevalence of home dialysis in
the UK, but not in the rest of Europe to anything like the same extent?
Why is limited care apparently replacing home dialysis in the USA?

In the UK, our socialized system of health care has undoubtedly played
an important part in promoting home dialysis, despite the initial tardy
response of the then Ministry of Health to demands for funding for this
form of treatment. The existence of the National Health Service has encouraged people to expect and demand health care as a right. This meant
that a vociferous demand for dialysis for patients with kidney failure could
be expected, and free treatment at that. Expectations were fulfilled. A key
question was to be how to provide this extremely expensive form of treatment for as many patients as possible.

The National Health Service had an inheritance of specialist and non-
specialist hospitals housed typically in cramped Victorian buildings in

inner-city areas without physical space for expansion. Health care was not high amongst the Government's priorities for spending, and the rate of spending on health care as a percentage of our gross national product was steadily slowing down[2]. Thus the climate was not ripe for the rapid growth of highly specialized new units. Home dialysis was apparently the only way that the demand for treatment could begin to be met. It was the only way that the small numbers of medical, nursing and technical staff skilled in dialysis techniques could hope to support a steadily growing population of patients. Luckily there was and is substantial evidence that the rehabilitation of home dialysis patients was more successful than that of hospital-based patients, and that the risk of hepatitis amongst patients and staff was dramatically reduced. And so was born the British taste for home dialysis.

In the USA, with its free-market system of health care and health insurance, another influence is felt in the development of patterns of treatment – that of financial incentives and disincentives. It has been suggested that the falling off of home dialysis during the years 1972–75 was as a result of the increase in limited-care units[1]. But what were the reasons for that growth? It is likely that it has been caused by the financial disincentive to the patient to dialyse at home (health insurance does not cover the entire cost of treatment), and by the financial advantage to the physician to have the patient dialyse in the limited care unit or hospital setting.

In neither the UK nor the USA can the needs of the patient at the time be said to be the prime consideration in determining the forms of treatment to be offered.

The economic good sense of putting resources primarily into home dialysis in the UK has been amply reinforced by evidence of the many practical advantages to the dialysis patient and his or her family. The relatively small number of renal units meant that the catchment area of each unit was wide. After their initial period of training, patients no longer had to travel long distances for treatment. They could dialyse as and when they liked, and could return to full-time work.

5.2 SOME PLANNING CONSIDERATIONS

Home dialysis has thus continued to be the main form of treatment offered in the UK as a matter of expediency. The staff of individual renal units have been encouraged by all the evidence suggesting the success of home dialysis, as far as the patients treated are concerned. But there has been little serious reference to the unmet regional and national need for dialysis. There has been little attempt to address in a practical way the problem of inequalities of distribution of dialysis facilities amongst different regions.

There has been little serious consideration of the changing needs of our existing population of patients already established on home dialysis.

In planning for future needs, it is essential that these three considerations are linked together since they have a circular relationship (Figure 5.1). The

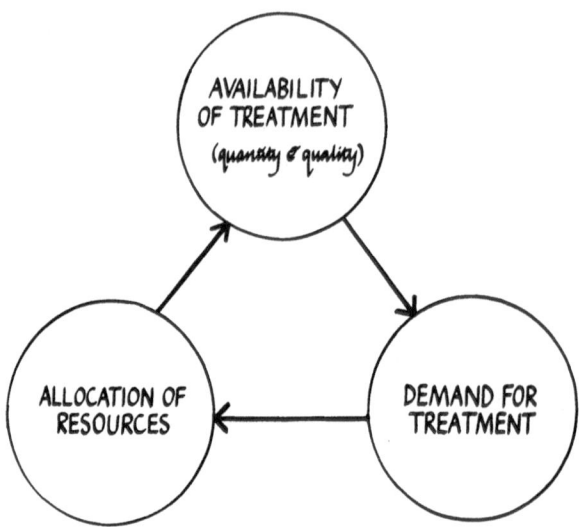

Figure 5.1   Planning considerations

demand for treatment is created by the current availability of treatment[3], i.e. local doctors are less likely to refer patients to hospitals with dialysis facilities if they feel that dialysis will not be available because of limited resources. But resources for the future are allocated all too often according to the existing demand. For example, the City and East London Area Health Authority plan for 1977–78 rightly describes the allocation by the North-East Thames Regional Health Authority for dialysis in the AHA as arbitrary[4]. The capital allocation for dialysis for 1977–78 of £150 000 was the same as it had been the previous year, without regard even for inflation – a cut in real terms of 17%!

If current availability, demand and allocation of resources are linked in this way, then it should be possible to use pressure for change in one area as a tool for influencing the other areas in a planned way. It is in this light that the need for and practicalities of a limited-care unit in Essex is examined starting with a survey of dialysis patients at the St. Leonard's/St. Bartholomew's Regional Renal Unit in Hackney in East London.

5.3   A SURVEY OF PATIENTS LIVING IN ESSEX

The patients at the St. Leonard's/St. Bartholomew's Renal Unit come from all over the North-East Thames Health Region, but are mainly concentrated in east London and south-east Essex. A few come from outside the Region. Currently there is a total of 72 patients established on home dialysis. The proportion of patients referred annually from Essex has increased from 33% in 1968 to 50% in 1976. A total of 40 patients from Essex has been established on home dialysis since 1968. The survey focuses on the experience of these 40 patients.

The renal unit offers a joint home dialysis and transplantation programme, but offers no facilities for regular limited-care or hospital-based dialysis. It is becoming increasingly clear that these facilities are inadequate to meet the changing needs of our patients.

As we gain confidence in our ability to train patients for home dialysis, so we develop a more catholic attitude towards patient selection. Patients now come on to the home dialysis programme who in earlier days would have been turned down because of their social, psychological or economic situation. We now have single patients who have no partner, and who dialyse entirely on their own. We have patients who are separated or divorced and patients who are single parents. We have immigrant patients who speak limited English and patients who have difficulty in reading.

Hand-in-hand with less stringent selection comes a galaxy of practical problems, the chief of which is bad housing, closely followed by low income, unemployment, and unstable family relationships.

5.4   HOUSING AND HOME DIALYSIS

East London and south-east Essex have a high density of local authority and Greater London Council housing. Council houses are allocated according to family size, and so council tenants will almost by definition not have a spare room. The St. Leonard's/St. Bartholomew's Renal Unit has always operated a policy of using only a spare room for dialysis, for reasons of hygiene (easier to keep clean), and for psychological reasons (easier to close the door and forget about dialysis). With the wider use of disposable artificial kidneys, automatic supply units with built-in washing-through mechanisms, and shorter hours of dialysis, this policy could change. However, the need for rehousing would not decrease dramatically, as rooms in many council houses and flats are cramped and dialysis in the sitting room or bedroom would still be unacceptable in many cases.

Of our 40 Essex patients, only 15 had rooms in their houses which were

TABLE 5.1   Home dialysis arrangements for 40 patients from Essex

Suitable room for conversion	15
Elaborate conversion, extension or portable cabin	9
Rehoused	15
No permanent solution	1
Total	40

suitable for conversion into dialysis treatment rooms (Table 5.1). Nine had expensive portable cabins, extensions to their houses, or elaborate conversions. Fifteen had to be rehoused by the local authority or Greater London Council. For one patient, an owner-occupier, there was no solution as his house was under planning blight because of a road scheme. Council housing was refused, and the patient is temporarily receiving what is rather inadequate dialysis on a portable dialysis machine.

Thus the solution for ten patients was extremely costly in initial capital outlay. Fifteen other patients had to endure the considerable domestic upheaval and worry of moving house, and frequently moving to a new neighbourhood, while travelling to the renal unit three times weekly for dialysis. Financial assistance with moving is only automatically forthcoming for patients claiming Supplementary Benefit – another hidden cost of NHS 'free' dialysis. Some patients have felt pressured by the renal unit into accepting larger council accommodation which they did not like, so that there would be no delay in starting home dialysis. This may have contributed to domestic and dialysis-related problems which occurred later.

5.5   LENGTH OF TIME BEFORE HOME DIALYSIS

Another factor worthy of consideration is the length of time it takes from the first dialysis at the renal unit to the first home dialysis. This is determined by two factors; the time taken to adapt the patient's home, and the patient's ability to dialyse. Adapting the home involves drawing up plans, seeking estimates, and carrying out the building work. The time taken will depend on the efficiency of the various public authorities involved, and the amount of bureaucratic red tape deemed necessary. The patient's ability to dialyse depends on having an adequate fistula, adequately controlled weight gains and blood pressure, a lack of other medical problems, competence in dialysis technique, and confidence in his or her own ability to dialyse. Competence and confidence will in turn be influenced by the staffing of the renal unit. At the same time as increasing numbers of patients are being accepted for dialysis each year (made possible by recycling of capital equipment), staffing levels are being frozen because of financial cutbacks. A lower staff/patient ratio leads to less concentrated teaching. Strain on the staff leads to rapid staff turnover, and patients cannot depend on having their accustomed teacher.

Table 5.2 Average length of time between first hospital dialysis and first home dialysis of 40 patients from Essex, according to home dialysis arrangement

Suitable room for conversion	7–8 months
Elaborate conversion, extension or portable cabin	8–9 months
Rehoused	10–11 months

Looking at the length of time between the first hospital and first home dialysis in the 40 Essex patients, there has been a general trend for this time to increase slightly between 1968 and 1976 (Table 5.2). If broken down according to whether the patient had to be rehoused or not, it can be seen that rehousing tends to prolong the time by 2–4 months.

5.6 THE CHANGING NEEDS

If the capital expense to the National Health Service, the expense to the patient in moving house, and inconvenience and expense of travelling anything up to 60 miles to the renal unit during training were the happy end of the story, our policy of home dialysis alone would be easily justified. But the happiest end to the story for many patients is successful kidney transplantation, and the removal of dialysis equipment from their homes. For patients who are not transplanted and are ageing, there may be increasing difficulty with access sites and additional medical complications, which will limit the possibility of continued home dialysis. The cumulative stress of home dialysis may cause social or psychological problems, which will also make home dialysis impossible. From these patients there will be an increasing demand for frequent and possibly permanent unit-based dialysis.

Table 5.3 shows how the circumstances of 17 patients have changed

TABLE 5.3 Changes in circumstances of 40 home dialysis patients in Essex

Successful transplants	7
Failed/failing transplants	4
Return to unit-based dialysis	3
Deaths	3
Unchanged	23
Total	40

since they were established on home dialysis. It is clear that for a sizable minority of patients, home dialysis cannot be a permanent solution.

5.7   THE NEED FOR LIMITED-CARE DIALYSIS

Taking into account the changing needs of our patients and the catchment area of the St. Leonard's/St. Bartholomew's Renal Unit, the evidence suggests a considerable and immediate need for an additional satellite dialysis unit in Essex, offering limited-care dialysis. Furthermore, the St. Leonard's/St. Bartholomew's Renal Unit does not have the monopoly of patients with chronic renal failure in Essex. The catchment area of The London Hospital Renal Unit is identical. The Royal Free Hospital Renal Unit is also in the North-East Thames Health Region and maintains some patients in Essex. The needs of these two units should also be taken into account, thus creating a regional facility for limited care.

Training in dialysis for the patient needs to take place at the parent-unit where there is medical and out-patient back-up. But once a patient has been trained, there is no reason why he or she should not dialyse in a limited-care setting, if home dialysis is not possible for some reason. Limited care would mean that the patient could either be totally auton-omous, or could receive assistance from staff in certain clearly defined areas, e.g. needling, machine preparation and clearing up.

A limited-care unit would offer a flexible solution to changing problems. Patients could use it in a variety of different situations. It could be the permanent base of those few Essex patients who are at present dialysing long-term or permanently in the hospital. It could be used as an interim measure for patients requiring rehousing or who suffer long delays in the completion of their home dialysis adaptations, but are otherwise self-sufficient in their treatment. This would save the patient money as well as time, since travelling expenses are only automatically refunded to patients who claim Supplementary Benefits. This can cause considerable hardship to patients who are at work or claiming other benefits. It might be used occasionally as a long-term solution for patients whose homes are particu-larly difficult to convert and who may be good candidates for transplanta-tion. Patients who had temporarily or permanently lost confidence in their ability to dialyse at home could use it. It could be used to give patients on 'holiday' a break from dialysing at home on their own.

The St. Leonard's/St. Bartholomew's Unit already offers this facility to home patients, but not one of the 11 patients who came into the Unit in 1977 for holiday dialysis came from Essex. Presumably, the distance, travelling time and expense involved cancel out the benefit for patients who live some distance away. It is probable therefore that there would be a considerable demand for holiday dialysis in an Essex limited-care unit.

5.8 SITING AND STRUCTURE

The flexible usage of such a unit should be reflected in its physical structure. A system of linked prefabricated units would be cheap and would allow for future expansion. The conversion of an existing disused building might also be considered. The siting of the unit would depend on the geographical distribution of the patients of all the renal units concerned, and should take carefully into account the question of ease of access by public transport. The Essex patients from the St. Leonard's/St. Bartholomew's Unit come mainly from south Essex, in the triangle formed between Basildon, Chelmsford and Southend-on-Sea (Figure 5.2). Since the smaller number of patients from north Essex travel the greatest distances, the siting of a limited-care unit in Chelmsford would seem practical.

The use of disposable dialysers and automatic supply units with built-in washing-through mechanisms would obviate the need for separate 'dirty' and 'clean' areas. It would also simplify the plumbing and drainage arrange-

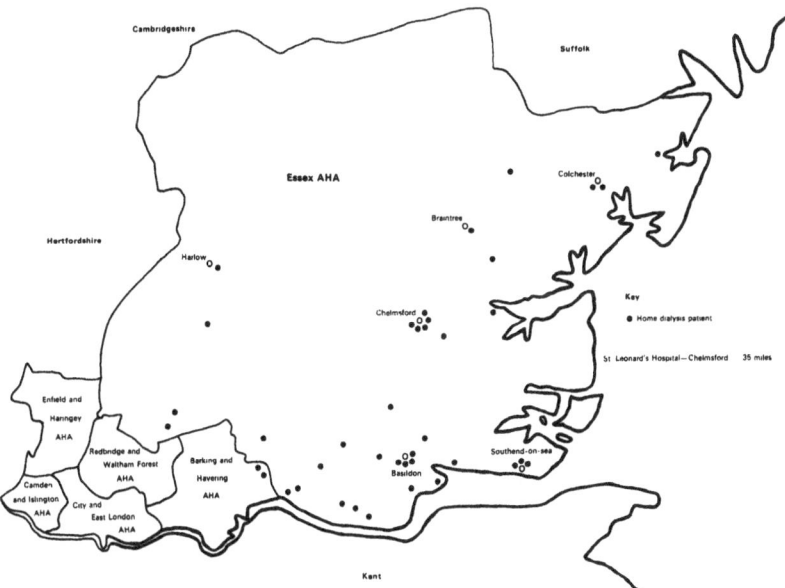

Figure 5.2 Distribution of home dialysis patients from St. Leonard's RDU living in Essex

ments. Armchairs rather than beds would allow a greater number of patients to dialyse in a smaller space, and would help discourage the patient from feeling that he or she was an invalid. Patients who had formerly dialysed at home might be especially prone to this.

The number of dialysis stations would depend finally on the projected regional need for limited-care dialysis. Four dialysis stations would allow 16 patients thrice-weekly dialysis, dialysing for 6-hour sessions, during the day and evening. The number of patients would increase to 24 if an overnight shift were included. Staffing considerations would also play a part in determining the size of the unit.

Besides the dialysis area, there should be space for storage of supplies and cleaning equipment, and WC, washing and changing facilities of a minimal kind. A living-room area with a small cooker where patients could prepare snacks could also serve as a staff room.

5.9 STAFFING AND WORKING HOURS

A unit with four dialysis stations could be staffed by Artificial Kidney Assistants (AKA), with one AKA in attendance at any one time. AKAs might staff the unit on a rotational basis from the parent units to prevent over-dependence on any one AKA, and prevent that AKA from becoming isolated. Technical back-up would come from the parent units. Technicians would do routine servicing and emergency call-outs as they do for home dialysis patients. Cleaning would be done by local domestic staff.

Patients would have to be responsible for their own drugs as if they were dialysing at home, to avoid the legal complications of the administration of drugs by AKAs. Patients would also keep their own dialysis records, and would attend the parent unit for routine medical examinations, unless facilities were developed for a renal out-patient clinic at a local hospital. The same would apply for routine urea and electrolyte blood tests, and hepatitis B antigen tests. The monitoring of patients and staff for hepatitis would need to be carefully organized, and a code of practice laid down for the unit.

A limited-care unit set up on this basis would represent a considerable challenge to the present piecemeal development of services for chronic renal failure. The considerations will be different in rural areas, but the same considerations could be readily applied to other urban areas of Britain.

5.10 CONCLUSION

When the National Health Service was reorganized in 1974, part of the aim was to provide regional budgets out of which comprehensive health services could be developed[5]. But there is little evidence that this is taking place either within individual regions, or amongst different regions. The policy of the Resource Allocation Working Party of redistribution of resources away from the four London regions and Merseyside serves only to spread the jam more thinly in a time of economic recession and cutbacks in public spending. The North-East Thames Regional Health Authority is the best served in the country as far as numbers of patients on long-term dialysis and numbers of weekly sessions by nephrologists are concerned. Yet even in this region, we are nowhere near treating the 33–40 patients per million population per year that it is estimated could benefit from long-term dialysis[6].

The setting up of a Regional Limited-Care Dialysis Unit would encourage local renal units to overcome their tendency to be isolated and insular. It would demand a serious attempt to assess the problem of the unmet need for dialysis. The presence of such a unit would encourage local doctors to refer patients with chronic renal failure to hospitals with dialysis facilities. Patients who today are dying because of doubts that the facility to treat them exists could be offered treatment. It would encourage the establishment of local renal out-patient clinics. Finally it would offer an important new type of care that would widen the spectrum of treatment available, to offer a more flexible and comprehensive service to people with chronic renal failure.

The correctness of asking for more resources in a field of medicine that already swallows up a large slice of the cake may be questioned, especially in a time of economic restraint. But conversely, if renal services are to be 'rationalized', it is our responsibility to make known the real needs of our patients. If we fail to, we will find ourselves not only with inadequate but inappropriate facilities.

References

1. Gurland, H. J., Brunner, F. P., Chantler, C., Jacobs, C., Schärer, K., Selwood, N. H., Spies, G. and Wing, A. J. (1976). Combined report on regular dialysis and transplantation in Europe, VI, 1975. *Transpl. Assoc.*, 13, 3
2. Central Statistical Office Annual Abstract of Statistics (1975). No. 112
3. Abel-Smith, B. (1976). *Value for Money in the Health Services.* Ch. 7 (London: Heinemann)

4. Area Plan 1977–78, The City and East London Area Health Authority (Teaching)
5. National Health Service Reorganisation Act (1973). Section 47 (London: HMSO)
6. Report of the Executive Committee of the Renal Association (1976). Distribution of nephrological services for adults in Great Britain. *Br. Med. J.*, 2, 903

DISCUSSION

Miss S. Taber: I would be interested in what members of the audience would feel about a limited-care unit without the nursing staff.

Mrs Deirdre E. Jones (London): One is very conditioned by what one is used to. It is the middleman between home dialysis and the hospital, which is the problem. We are very happy to let the patients do everything at home and to leave the responsibility to relatives. It is hard to visualize this in-between area. Why should a well-trained properly-educated Artificial Kidney Assistant (AKA) not manage such a situation? One gets concerned as much for the AKA's welfare as for the patients' in the situation when something goes wrong. It is a question of how much responsibility can be put on to the patient, and how much, possibly, on to the AKA. It is an area that has not been clearly defined. It is disheartening that nothing has come from the DHSS symposium on this. Hopefully the RCN group will come up with something. However, we have discussed this kind of area for years, and nothing really concrete is coming forward as guidelines.

Taber: What came out of the DHSS symposium was that we are to go back to the guidelines that were issued in 1966, or so the RCN delegation that went to the Department of Health was told. So we are back on the 1966 guidelines.

B. H. B. Robinson (Birmingham): We have been planning a similar unit and we would aim to get patients trained to a home dialysis standard, running their own dialysis, perhaps with the help of their relatives. All that the attendant would do would be to make sure that they clear up after themselves. If we look too much at guidelines and at who shall be responsible for what we shall rapidly find that we are running another hospital-type set up.

J. M. Bone (Liverpool): We are at the bottom of the league table as regards resources and the provision of facilities and we have no official hospital dialysis unit where we can support patients awaiting transplantation. We have been looking at limited care to support patients, primarily for transplantation in the first instance. If the transplant fails the patients will be back to limited care, or we might be able to arrange home haemodialysis. For the moment we have taken our proposals as far as we can. In the present financial climate the draught blows quite cold and there has been a call for savings of a million pounds in the District, so it is likely that we are in something of a limbo. Hopefully things might improve in the next financial year, and we might have the resources.

A. C. Kennedy (Glasgow): What thought has been given to the precise siting of the proposed unit? Would it be in the grounds of a hospital, or not?

Miss Rosenthal: It could be, but that is not necessary.

Kennedy: If it is in the grounds of a hospital, it will be difficult to get the Authority to stand back and not impose responsibilities, such as insisting on a qualified nurse being in attendance.

Rosenthal: It would be a matter of weighing up the advantages and the disadvantages. An existing but disused building in the grounds of a hospital might be available for conversion.

Kennedy: But, with respect, that would become a part of that hospital.

Miss Mary E. Selsby (London): I could not agree more with Professor Kennedy. I do not think that such a unit should be in the hospital grounds. That could only lead to problems.

I can see problems in using such a unit for patients who are waiting to be rehoused. Patients who have been in hospital for any length of time often lose the incentive to undertake home haemodialysis and I can see similar dangers arising with limited care.

Rosenthal: I can see the point, but in my own experience most patients want to get home. They do not enjoy being in a hospital setting. If the general atmosphere was superior to a hospital that might make a difference.

W. R. Cattell (London): Limited care has to be *limited* care. The patients must be self-sufficient dialysers and it then becomes a question of whether they dialyse in the unit or at home. I do not think that that really matters.

I would not be too unhappy about an individual who was permanently on self-supervised dialysis in a satellite limited-care unit if that was what he elected to do.

We ought to have some flexibility about this. The patient who requires treatment and who is capable of self-treatment could be treated in his own home, if suitable, or in a truly limited-care setting.

Selsby: But then such a unit would not be used for the patient awaiting rehousing.

Cattell: It might, but then the patient elects to have a house prepared. If there is any doubt about him waiting one would not waste the money.

6

Experience in self-care and limited-care haemodialysis in 340 patients
A. W. Siemsen

6.1 INTRODUCTION

Good preventive medical programmes and increased ability to resolve acute medical problems have resulted in a longer life expectancy and an increased incidence of chronic medical illness. The rate of dying varies from one person to another but is basically a function of the ageing process and superimposed disease. As part of the ageing process, there are concerns of adaptation to loneliness and various physical and mental infirmities[1]. In this setting the patient may have additional problems such as hypertension, coronary artery disease, cerebral vascular disease, diabetes mellitus or malignant processes.

The new technologies of haemodialysis and transplantation have made it possible to sustain life past the point where it would have normally ended. However, there remains a degree of uncertainty about their long-term effects on the body and the burdens which they place on families and societies. We have little understanding of the nature of uraemic toxins, which characteristically produce neuro-behavioural manifestations. Because of multifaceted patient and societal concerns created by increasing chronic medical illness and the new technologies, we must carefully evaluate all of the alternate treatment programmes so that the most reasonable course of action may be determined by patient and physician.

Patient selection to determine who will benefit from these treatment modalities can probably only be morally and legally justified if all patients with equal degrees of medical illness are chosen at random, such as by a lottery[2]. We have never practised patient selection because we have been unable to predict which patients will do well on dialysis and which will have serious medical and emotional problems. Flipping a coin would have been as accurate as our predictions.

To make an informed, competent decision of method and modality of care, the uraemic patient must be removed from his uraemic environment by dialysis or transplantation, have an opportunity to experience the nature of the treatment programmes, and have any emotional or adjustment problems evaluated and treated. Thus, nearly all patients not moribund from non-uraemic causes should be dialysed for a trial period so that they might adequately evaluate the situation themselves.

Our patients were offered: (a) living related transplantation if a suitable donor was available, (b) self-care dialysis at home or in an outpatient facility as near their home as possible or (c) limited-care dialysis in an outpatient facility near a hospital. If cadaveric transplantation was desired, the patient was placed on the waiting list. All self-dialysis patients entered a special teaching programme. Language barriers were not a contraindication to self-dialysis training. Home patients were required to have a back-up member who was taught by the patient. Re-use of the dialyser was routinely taught although some home patients subsequently discontinued this practice. The staff-to-patient ratio in the self-care facility was 1:5, as not all patients were totally independent. However, most were able to set up the dialyser, perform their dialysis and clean the dialyser. Many required assistance in placing the fistula needles. Re-use of the dialyser was utilized in all self-care facilities. The self-care facilities were commonly used by home patients when the back-up member desired a holiday. They were also used as an intermediate facility for home patients to gain confidence away from the centre before dialysis was actually done at home. This seemed to be particularly important in more remote areas. The ratio of staff to patients in the limited-care facilities was 1:3, as total care was provided by nurses or technicians. In Hawaii there are dialysis facilities located on three neighbour islands, as well as on Oahu in the State of Hawaii and in Majuro and Guam in Micronesia. Home patients were located on islands throughout the State and in Tahiti.

6.2 STATUS OF SELF-DIALYSIS TEACHING

Of the 349 patients admitted to our programme between 1 October 1968 and 30 November 1976, nine chose immediate living related transplantation or expired with less than one month of dialysis. The remaining 340 patients were retrospectively divided into three groups based on the age at initiation of dialysis: (a) 7–44 years (mean age 30.8 years), (b) 45–59 years (mean age 52.4 years), and (c) 60–80 years (mean age 66.5 years). Table 6.1 shows that 241 patients entered the self-dialysis teaching programme (SDTP) and the remainder were treated in the limited-care facilities (LCF). In the entire programme, 70.9% entered the self-dialysis teaching programme. This ranged from 79.1% in the younger age groups to 58.6% in the older age group. With advancing age a greater percentage entered the limited-care facilities.

TABLE 6.1   Status of self-dialysis teaching, 1 October 1968 – 30 November 1976

	Number of patients		
Age (years)	Entered LCF	Entered SDTP	Total
7–44	31 (20.9%)	117 (79.1%)	148
45–59	39 (32.0%)	83 (68.0%)	122
60–80	29 (41.4%)	41 (58.6%)	70
Entire programme	99 (29.1%)	241 (70.9%)	340

LCF – Limited-care facility
SDTP – Self-dialysis teaching programme

TABLE 6.2   Status of self-dialysis teaching, 1 October 1968 – 30 November 1976

| Age (years) | % Male | | |
	Entered LCF	Entered SDTP	Entire age group
7–44	61.3%	53.8%	55.4%
45–59	76.9%	57.8%	63.9%
60–80	69.0%	75.6%	72.9%
Entire programme	69.7%	58.9%	62.0%

Table 6.2 characterizes these groups by the percentage that were males. It can be noted that the percentage of males in each group increased from 55.4% in the youngest age group to 72.9% in the older age group with 62% of the entire dialysis population being male. The percentage of males entering the teaching programme tended to parallel the increased percentage of males in each age group. Nevertheless, more males were treated by limited-care dialysis (69.7%) than entered the teaching programme (58.9%). Thus, females tended to be more interested in self-dialysis than males.

TABLE 6.3   Status of self-dialysis teaching, 1 October 1968 – 30 November 1976

| Age (years) | % Diabetics | | |
	Entered LCF	Entered SDTP	Entire age group
7–44	19.4%	8.5%	10.8%
45–59	46.2%	25.3%	32.0%
60–80	75.9%	24.4%	45.7%
Entire programme	46.5%	17.0%	25.6%

The incidence of diabetes mellitus in each group is depicted in Table 6.3. The diagnosis of diabetes mellitus was made in 25.6% of those in the entire dialysis population. The frequency of this diagnosis increased with advancing age from 10.8% in the youngest group to 45.7% in the oldest age group. There was clearly a greater percentage of diabetics who required care in the limited-care programmes (46.5%) as compared with those entering the self-dialysis teaching programme (17%). This was explainable by the greater incidence of medical complications, including severe cerebral and coronary vascular disease, as well as blindness, in the limited-care group.

6.3 INITIAL MODALITY OF SELF-DIALYSIS

Table 6.4 subdivides the ultimate destination of those who entered the self-dialysis teaching programme into home and self-care facilities (SCF). This group does not total 241, the number entering the teaching programme, because of transplantation, deaths and those remaining in the teaching unit

TABLE 6.4 Initial modality of self-dialysis

Age (years)	Number of patients		
	Home	SCF	Total
7–44	59 (50.9%)	57 (49.1%)	116
45–59	43 (52.4%)	39 (47.6%)	82
60–80	12 (40.0%)	18 (60.0%)	30
Entire programme	114 (50.0%)	114 (50.0%)	228

as of 30 November 1976. In analysing the same three age groups, it was found that 50.9% of the younger age group went home; whereas this was only accomplished in 40% of the older group. Of the total group entering the teaching programme, 50% went home and 50% were treated in a self-care facility. The usual reasons a patient did not go home were lack of a back-up member, unstable psychological problems at home or inadequate housing. Thus, our initial experience (Tables 6.1 and 6.4) suggests that 30% of the patients on chronic maintenance dialysis would require limited-care dialysis while 35% could be treated at home and 35% in a self-care facility. These numbers are slightly biased as there is no home dialysis in Micronesia.

The percentage of males in each of the self-dialysis teaching age groups is summarized in Table 6.5. In general, and particularly in the middle age

TABLE 6.5 Initial modality of self-dialysis

Age (years)	% Males		
	Home	SCF	Entire age group
7–44	50.8%	56.1%	53.4%
45–59	46.5%	69.2%	57.3%
60–80	75.0%	72.2%	73.3%
Entire programme	51.8%	63.2%	57.4%

TABLE 6.6   Initial modality of self-dialysis

| Age (years) | % Diabetic | | |
	Home	SCF	Entire age group
7–44	8.5%	8.8%	8.6%
45–59	18.6%	25.6%	22.0%
60–80	33.3%	22.2%	26.7%
Entire programme	14.9%	16.7%	15.8%

group, a greater percentage of females were dialysing at home than males. Table 6.6 demonstrates that the diabetics who entered the self-dialysis teaching programme were eventually divided equally between the home and self-care programmes.

It is important to consider transfers from the initial programmes which the patients entered. Table 6.7 shows that 14.5% of those taught self-dialysis eventually entered other programmes. The highest rate of transfer occurred in the older age group. The usual transfer of a home-care patient was to a self-care facility although, before the 21 home patients transferred, they had accumulated 357 patient-months of experience at home. The most common cause of transfer was the magnitude of the emotional burden on the back-up member in the family. Multiple back-up members clearly aided successful home dialysis. When the back-up member was the husband, there were more transfers than when the back-up member was the wife.

The transfers from self-care facilities were generally to a limited-care facility, although two patients eventually went home. However, before the eight patients transferred, they had experienced 90 patient-months in self-care dialysis. The usual cause of the self-care transfers was increasing medical complications which had arisen on dialysis, such as poor cardiac output, serious cardiac arrhythmia and cerebral vascular accidents.

TABLE 6.7   Self-dialysis transfers

| Age (years) | Number of patients | | | % of those taught for age group |
	Home	SCF	SDTP	
7–44	13	0	0	11.1%
45–59	6	2	0	9.6%
60–80	2	6	6	34.1%
Entire programme	21	8	6	14.5%

There were six patients (2.5%) who were unable to complete the self-dialysis teaching programme and had to be transferred to a limited-care facility. These patients were all in the older age group. Of the 35 patient transfers, 31.4% were diabetic, as compared with 17% entering the teaching programme, and 62.8% were male, as compared with 58.9% entering the teaching programme.

6.4 MORBIDITY AND MORTALITY

Any treatment programme must initially be evaluated from the perspective of morbidity and mortality. Table 6.8 shows that our data is based on 7824 patient-months or 652 patient-years of experience. The largest experience

TABLE 6.8   Patient-months of experience, 1 October 1968 – 30 November 1976

Age (years)	LCF	SDT	Home	SCF	Entire age group
7–44	965	107	1669	1379	4120
45–59	686	114	1128	572	2500
60–80	702	48	182	272	1204
Entire programme	2353	269	2979	2223	7824

of 2979 patient-months was accumulated in home dialysis. The younger age group with 4120 patient-months was larger than the other two age groups. The index of morbidity chosen was number of hospital days. This data is presented in Table 6.9. This was corrected to hospital days per 1000 patient-months of experience so that the various treatment modalities and age groups could be compared.

TABLE 6.9   Hospital days per 1000 patient-months of experience

Age (years)	LCF	SDT	Home	SCF	Entire age group
7–44	3258	1878	747	1004	1451
45–59	4729	1316	1007	1420	2137
60–80	4199	938	1582	2412	3270
Entire programme	3968	1472	897	1283	1950

In the entire dialysis programme, our patients had been hospitalized 1950 days per 1000 patient-months of dialysis, or these patients were in the hospital for 1 day out of every 15.4 days on dialysis. Home patients had the lowest number of inpatient days with 1 per 33.4 days on dialysis and limited-care, the highest with 1 day out of 7.6 days on dialysis. The lowest incidence of hospitalization was in the younger age group on home dialysis with 1 hospital day out of every 40.2 days on dialysis. There were increasing hospital days associated with advancing age. The most common cause of hospitalization was related to vascular access.

The number of hospital days per admission are shown in Table 6.10. This averaged 10.1 days for the entire programme and increased with advancing age.

TABLE 6.10   Hospital days per admission

Age (years)	LCF	SDT	Home	SCF	Entire age group
7–44	9.1	6.9	7.7	8.3	8.5
45–59	12.5	6.8	9.5	8.8	10.8
60–80	12.2	5.6	9.9	15.6	12.3
Entire programme	11.0	6.7	8.6	9.5	10.1

The cumulative survival curves for diabetics and non-diabetics is given in Table 6.11. The non-diabetic survival curve in our experience was intermediate between living related and cadaveric transplantation. A more

TABLE 6.11   Haemodialysis cumulative survival

Years	Non-diabetic (%) ($n = 253$)	Diabetic (%) ($n = 87$)
0.25	93.9	98.8
0.5	91.6	88.7
1.0	87.5	74.3
2.0	80.6	53.8
3.0	70.8	33.5
4.0	61.2	23.2
5.0	59.1	
6.0	51.7	

sensitive index of mortality is the number of deaths per 1000 patient-months of experience. Table 6.12 shows that the mortality for the entire programme was 12.8 deaths per 1000 patient-months of experience. The mortality was 14.0 for males and 10.8 for females per 1000 patient-months of experience. Like morbidity, mortality increased with advancing age and was highest in the limited-care group.

TABLE 6.12   Mortality per 1000 patient-months of experience

Age (years)	LCF	SDT	Home	SCF	Entire age group
7–44	12.4	—	6.0	3.6	6.6
45–59	29.2	—	12.4	12.2	16.4
60–80	32.8	20.8	22.0	14.7	26.6
Entire group	23.4	3.7	9.4	7.2	12.8

If one analyses the data for morbidity (Table 6.9), it can be noted that the number of hospital days for limited-care patients was 3.1–4.4 times greater than for self-care or home patients. If one analyses the data for mortality (Table 6.12), it is apparent that deaths for the limited-care patients were 2.5–3.2 times greater than for home or self-care patients. These comparisons should not lead to a conclusion that limited-care dialysis is adverse. The limited-care patients are older, have a higher incidence of diabetes mellitus and other medical complications, and reflect a life-plan in which many patients, initially treated at home or in a self-care programme, eventually required total patient care.

6.5 RECENT TRENDS

The data presented was a total experience over the past 8 years. There are some important recent trends to be considered. Table 6.13 shows that the percentage of home patients progressively rose through 30 June 1973. In July of 1973, the 92nd Congress enacted Public Law 92–603 which substantially relieved the financial burden of end-stage renal disease patients; however, it contained several disincentives to home dialysis. It can be noted that the percentage of patients at home has progressively decreased since that time. The absolute number of patients going home is shown in

TABLE 6.13   Modality of dialysis

Date	Home (%)	SCF (%)	LCF (%)
30/6/71	40	18	42
30/6/72	40	24	36
30/6/73	49	21	30
30/6/74*	46	26	28
30/6/75	39	35	26
30/6/76	25	46	29

* Date funding acted against home dialysis

TABLE 6.14   Absolute number of new patients entering a programme

Date	Home	SCF	LCF
30/6/71	12	7	2
30/6/72	12	9	2
30/6/73	15	10	5
30/6/74*	7	29	11
30/6/75	8	24	14
30/6/76	3	47	21

* Date funding acted against home dialysis

Table 6.14. The absolute number of patients going home rose until enactment of the legislation and has since progressively decreased. In this programme, where there has been no change in the number of diabetics or medically more complicated patients accepted, it suggests that other factors such as loss of incentives or family burdens may be operational. The percentage and absolute number of patients entering self-care facilities has dramatically increased. The upward changes in the limited-care programme are less marked.

6.6 SOCIETAL CONCERNS

Through our advancing technology we can now prolong the life of a patient with end-stage renal disease. The new technology carries with it degrees of uncertainty and risk. It may produce severe emotional, physical and financial burdens on the patients and their families. The dissipation of tremendous resources causes society to debate the degree of benefit conferred on one group as compared to the burdens borne by another. Each society must make value judgements based on its goals and allocate resources appropriately to such things as building roads, subsidizing symphonies, combating unemployment, fighting wars, supporting end-stage renal disease, etc. If these resources are infinite, we could dialyse patients in posh surroundings with maximum services and conveniences. If resources are limited, as they are in our programme, we must consider more efficient forms of dialysis at home or in self-care facilities where cost, in our experience, can be reduced by 70% and 40% respectively. These reductions in cost ignore payment of the back-up member at home and require dialyser re-use. There may be patients who desire transfer out of home dialysis because of emotional stresses and burdens on the family, or patients in self-care facilities who develop medical complications which require limited-care dialysis. As the technology continues to advance and the societal constraints increase, we will probably develop an inverse relationship between scientific medicine and freedom of therapeutic choice[3].

Our self-care facility at Majuro in the Marshall Islands has dialysed 10 patients for three years at a location 2400 miles from Honolulu. This unit is operated only by nurses without a nephrologist in attendance. Wireless communication usually takes 24 hours or longer. The morbidity and mortality of this facility has been no different from our closer units. A nephrologist does visit the atoll every 4–5 months to evaluate the progress of patients. Complications occurring on dialysis are managed in Honolulu. Further cost reduction can be obtained by increased utilization of our nursing staff.

The public and our nursing personnel are well aware of the recent medical advances. We must constantly evaluate them as to the nature of chronic illness. We must dispel the notion that going to a doctor automatically offers the potential of a restored optimal state of health[4]. Patients on dialysis are not restored to their usual state of health which existed prior to the onset of uraemia. This frequently leads to frustration on the part of the nursing staff because there may be no dramatic improvement in the patient from one dialysis to another. A psychiatric nurse clinician plays a vital role in helping the staff to become more aware of their own feelings and that of their patients.

The major emerging moral, legal and medical concern is under what circumstances can dialysis be discontinued. The role of the informed competent adult and the guardian in the decision-making process requires further study.

Thus, with increasing chronic illness and advancing technology, we must constantly examine two spheres of interaction: medical and societal. How much of the burden should be borne by the patient and how much by society? We should tailor the dialysis to the patient needs in so far as possible within the limits of the burdens tolerated by society. We must examine all of the alternative solutions for the patients, their families and their society. Only in this way can we come up with the most reasonable course of action. The confidence of our patients and our society depends on our ability to handle them correctly.

References

1. Williams, R. H. (1969). Our role in the generation, modification and termination of life. *Arch. Intern. Med.*, **124**, 215
2. Dukeminier, J. and Sanders, D. (1971). Legal problems in allocation of scarce medical resources. *Arch. Inter. Med.*, **127**, 1133
3. Kountz, S. L. (1975). The effect of bioscience and technological momentum on the surgical treatment of chronic illness. *Surgery*, **77**, 735
4. Teschan, P. E. (1970). On the pathogenesis of uremia. *Am. J. Med.*, **48**, 671

DISCUSSION

A. M. Martin (Sunderland): Given Dr Siemsen's large experience with haemodialysis in diabetics, does he agree with the suggestion that heparinization accelerates the onset of blindness?

Siemsen: To give a scientific answer to that question I would need records going back over a period of time and I do not have that information. We have no peritoneal experience at this point; we are starting. We are starting largely because in diabetics there are problems of access, and at that point in time we shall start that study.

However, I believe that there is a consensus of opinion among nephrologists in the US today that heparin does aggravate failing vision in diabetics.

R. J. Winney (Edinburgh): Dr Siemsen seems to have a high incidence of diabetics. Were they all insulin-dependent diabetics since this may affect the complication rates?

Siemsen: They were not all insulin-requiring diabetics. However, I should point out that in Hawaii, and particularly in the Pacific Basin, there is an increased incidence of diabetes. The best statistics on this are obtainable from the Atomic Energy Commission. They have carried out a study and there is a higher incidence of diabetes.

Mrs Deirdre E. Jones (London): May we have a brief rundown on how the home training is approached.

Siemsen: We have a language problem and almost all the teaching is done by illustration. Most people can be taught to read numbers and we put numbers on all the switches. A great deal is 'watch monkey, do monkey' and a lot of teaching is done that way, with some of it done conventionally, where the subject is suitable, using illustrations, and the nurse doing the teaching. It is all on a one-to-one basis.

Jones: With how much relative involvement?

Siemsen: The patient is first taught to dialyse himself, and the patient then teaches the back-up member. The patient should be the prime mover.

A. C. Kennedy (Glasgow): I was interested to hear Dr Siemsen say that he considered that he had limited financial resources. All things are relative!

Siemsen: It took us two years of heavy lobbying to get funds from the State. It took an immense amount of time and energy before we were eventually successful. We have a pact with the legislature that we will keep the costs down and they will keep the patients alive, but they do watch it closely.

Kennedy: Given Dr Siemsen's experience of dialysing patients of 75, 80, 84 years of age, with many other physical problems, has he any doubts about the wisdom of doing this?

Siemsen: No, not at all. The gravest question that arises in my mind is because of the complications of diabetes. With vascular access problems, prolonged hospitalization, pain for the patient from repeated vascular procedures, loss of extremities unrelated to the vascular procedures, and disease, one must ask oneself how meaningful this life is.

Kennedy: Which is what I am asking.

Siemsen: But it is meaningful to that patient. Physicians might ask themselves whether it is meaningful to them, but it is meaningful to that patient and it is meaningful to that family.

J. M. Bone (Liverpool): One comment on the use of terms. Problems will arise in the future when we relate limited-care facilities to self-care facilities as there are at least two other terms on the horizon, one of them minimal-care, which is a slightly different aspect. However, Dr Siemsen uses the term 'limited-care' for what we would call hospital dialysis and he uses 'self-care' for what we would probably call limited-care dialysis. There is a spectrum of care between the hospital and the home and very different patients will require to be slotted into it depending on their circumstances.

Our use of limited-care, or our intended use of limited-care, will be for transplant support with a high turnover, and in these circumstances a staff ratio of five to one is probably adequate. But the patient who had a rejected kidney, who was rehabilitated and was back on self-care dialysis could probably go out to the periphery, not necessarily to his home, but perhaps to a health centre or to a facility nearby to a district general hospital, which would be total self-care.

There is a problem with terms.

Siemsen: When the original paper was presented in 1972, the term 'limited-care' was used for what would now be called self-care. Where we have acute renal failure and a critically ill patient, the ratio is usually one to one. Limited-care is the next step down, the stable maintenance patient, where we can use the ratio of one to three. That is limited, and not what it was. We then have a teaching programme to do self-care, either at home, or in a special self-care facility, where we try to get the patients as near totally independent as is possible.

That is how we are now defining it.

Unidentified speaker: I believe that Dr Siemsen said that he took people on to dialysis for a trial period and that they could withdraw. In the total number of cases, how many have asked to withdraw?

Siemsen: None. However, I believe the time is coming when someone will walk in and say that they are tired of the regime, that the burden is getting too great, and that they want to stop.

We have had problems making decisions, not where the patient wanted out, but where the patient was stroked out, deeply comatose, still had brainwaves but was not opening his eyes or responding, still had reflexes, and my inclination was to discontinue dialysis. In that one particular set of circumstances I was threatened with a law suit. Under such circumstances there should be ways to stop dialysis.

Our biggest area of concern now is how we are to stop.

W. R. Cattell (London): The implication earlier was that we must move towards less skilled people being available to deliver the care, and that doctors are not needed, probably nurses are not needed, and so on. This raises implications of medico-legal responsibility. I do not know about Honolulu, but in the US there are certainly problems with people suing the doctor on hand. In the limited-care situation, how would medical personnel cover themselves against being sued?

Siemsen: Most patients want to go home, or to be near their homes, and they are grateful for the opportunity to have what they are doing thoroughly explained to them.

Apart from that, I believe that one has to be a Martin Luther King and take a chance.

Cattell: Is there any legal indemnity, some kind of process for protection of those involved? Do the patients give some undertaking?

Siemsen: The limited-care facilities are all located in hospital grounds, but that is because back-up would then be on hand. We do not yet provide self-care, i.e. like at home, although that will have to come.

A. L. G. Moss (Nottingham): As a social worker I probably see things from a slightly different perspective. I was most interested in the description of the social and non-medical problems which are most important, and I tried to relate to something said by an earlier speaker to what we have been saying about limited-care. For several of the patients whom I come across their main need is to be able to dialyse in another situation apart from their own home, and in the UK it is too expensive for them to do it in hospital. I would see limited-care fulfilling that need. I maintain, and many of the patients maintain, that we ask too much of them to cope with the burden of home dialysis. It is a small percentage, but it is very important to that small percentage.

Siemsen: How many cases has Mr Moss seen where dialysis has driven a couple to divorce?

Moss: Not many personally, but I have come across cases that are on the brink, and my colleagues have also come across such cases.

Siemsen: In such circumstances it is probably best to bring the patient out of self-care facilities and to try to preserve that marriage.

Moss: Which is what I am suggesting. My point is that in the UK patients are asked to take on the burden of home dialysis. I grant that that is mainly because there is no other alternative, but patients are told that they must dialyse at home, and there is an assumption that patients and their relatives must accept that regardless. I am suggesting that that assumption is wrong.

Siemsen: I would say that too.

SECTION THREE

Some Clinical Problems
Chairman:
J. S. Cameron

7

Hypertension
J. D. Briggs

7.1 MECHANISM OF HYPERTENSION

Blood pressure commonly rises as chronic renal failure advances to the point where regular dialysis is needed to maintain life[1]. Sodium and renin have often been invoked in the pathogenesis of hypertension, and once dialysis has been initiated, it is possible to influence these two factors independently, the former by dialysis and the latter by bilateral neph-

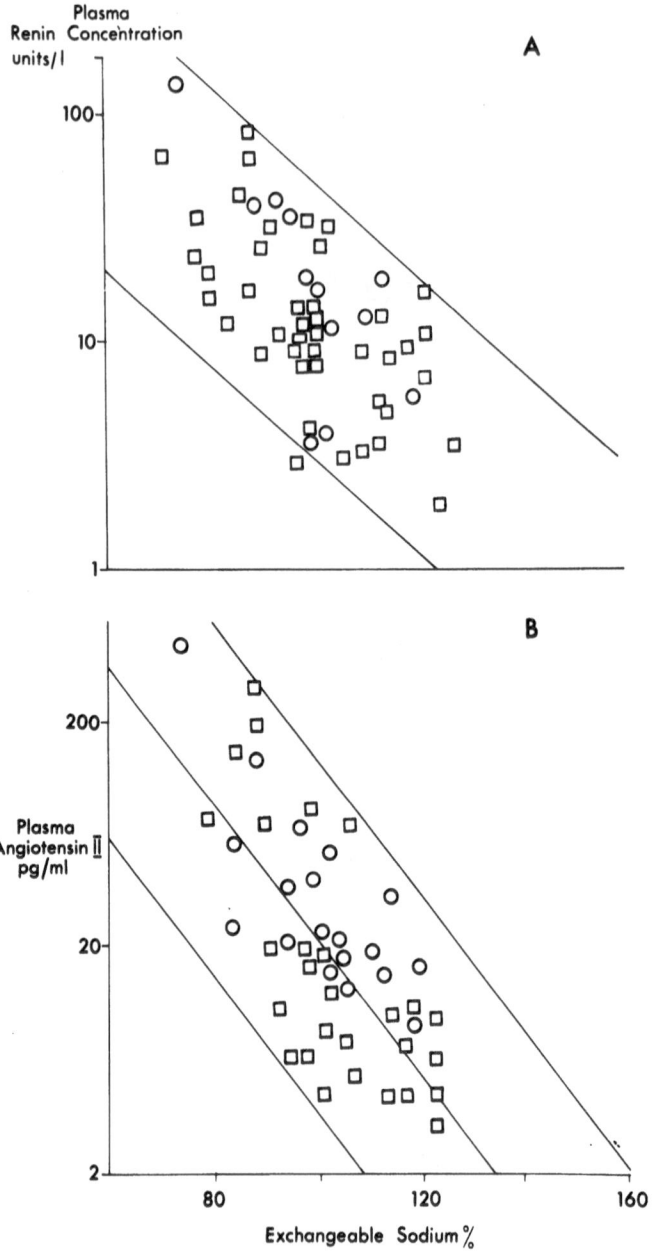

Figure 7.1   Relationship of exchangeable sodium to plasma renin (A) and to plasma angiotensin II (B) in normotensive patients with (O) and without (□) chronic renal failure

rectomy. The ability to do this has led to intensive study of hypertension in this situation.

Although excess sodium can raise blood pressure, the effect is variable and a consistent relationship between blood pressure and the level of exchangeable or plasma sodium is not commonly found in hypertensive patients[2]. Renin has a pressor effect through its active product, angiotensin II. There is, however, no close relationship between blood pressure and plasma renin in most types of hypertension[2]. By contrast, if one examines sodium and renin together, some positive relationships emerge and one cannot consider a role for sodium in hypertension in isolation from a role

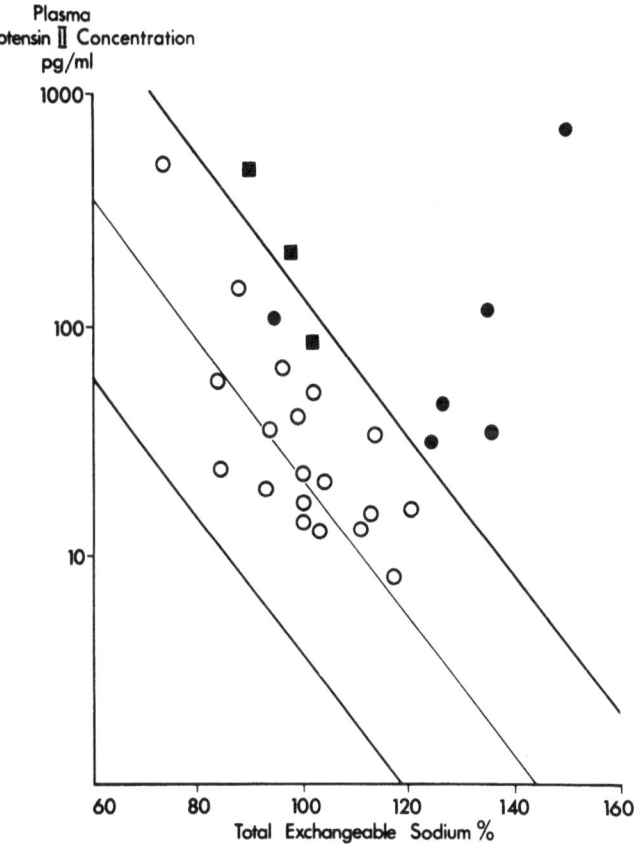

Figure 7.2 Relationship of exchangeable sodium to plasma angiotensin II in chronic renal failure patients with normal (O) and elevated (●) blood pressure. Also shown is the relationship for patients with malignant hypertension without renal failure (■)

for renin or vice versa. Figure 7.1 demonstrates the inverse relationship which exists between exchangeable sodium and both plasma renin and angiotensin II in normotensive patients with and without renal failure. As plasma renin and angiotensin II levels correlate very well in this situation, the inverse relationship with exchangeable sodium is virtually identical for each. In contrast to normotensive patients, those with hypertension and renal failure have high plasma angiotensin II levels in relation to exchangeable sodium (Figure 7.2). If the blood pressure can be restored to normal either by dialysis or bilateral nephrectomy, the abnormally high plasma angiotensin II levels will fall back to within the range in relation to exchangeable sodium which is seen in normotensive patients (Figure 7.3). Patients who are normotensive before treatment have plasma angiotensin II levels which are initially within the normal range in relation to exchangeable sodium and which remains in this range following dialysis or bilateral nephrectomy (Figure 7.3).

It is generally agreed that there are two forms of hypertension in chronic

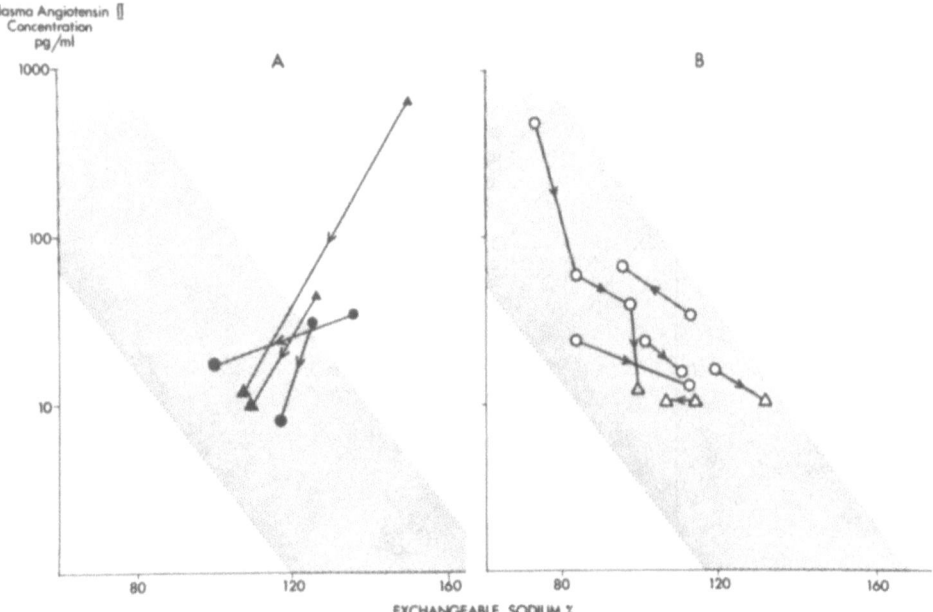

Figure 7.3   Relationship of exchangeable sodium to plasma angiotensin II. In panel A are four patients with chronic renal failure and hypertension before and after restoration of blood pressure to normal by dialysis (●) or bilateral nephrectomy (▲). In panel B are five patients with chronic renal failure without hypertension before and after dialysis (○) or bilateral nephrectomy (△)

renal failure, the more common controllable by dialysis, and an infrequent form which is unresponsive to dialysis[3]. In the former type, the relationship between plasma renin and exchangeable sodium is more horizontal than in normotensive subjects[3], as illustrated diagrammatically in Figure 7.4. This

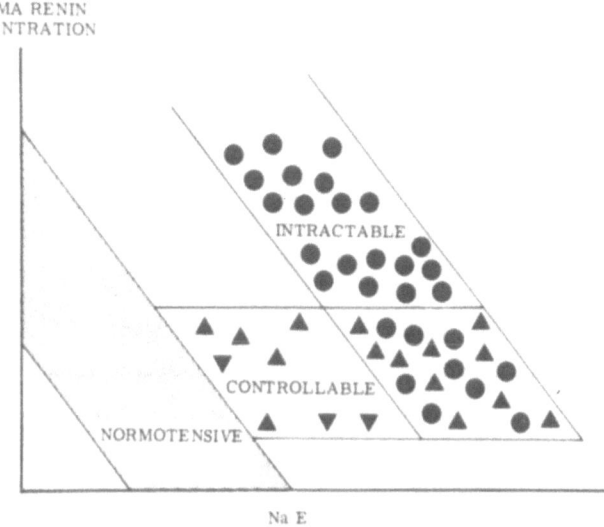

Figure 7.4 Diagrammatic representation of the relationship of exchangeable sodium (NaE) to plasma renin in chronic renal failure patients with controllable (▲) and intractable (●) hypertension

form of hypertension could arise if renin release were unresponsive to changes in sodium balance. There is supporting evidence for this in that the rise of plasma renin in patients of this type is relatively small during deprivation of dietary sodium or during sodium and water depleting dialysis treatments[4]. By contrast, in the intractable form of hypertension, plasma renin is abnormally raised in relation to exchangeable sodium, and remains so at all levels of exchangeable sodium (Figure 7.4). In these patients one would expect that an attempt to reduce blood pressure by sodium depletion would lead to a marked rise in plasma renin and such changes have in fact been demonstrated[4]. Figure 7.5 clearly illustrates the difference in renin response to dialysis in the two groups of patients. In the five patients with intractable hypertension, plasma renin rose in response

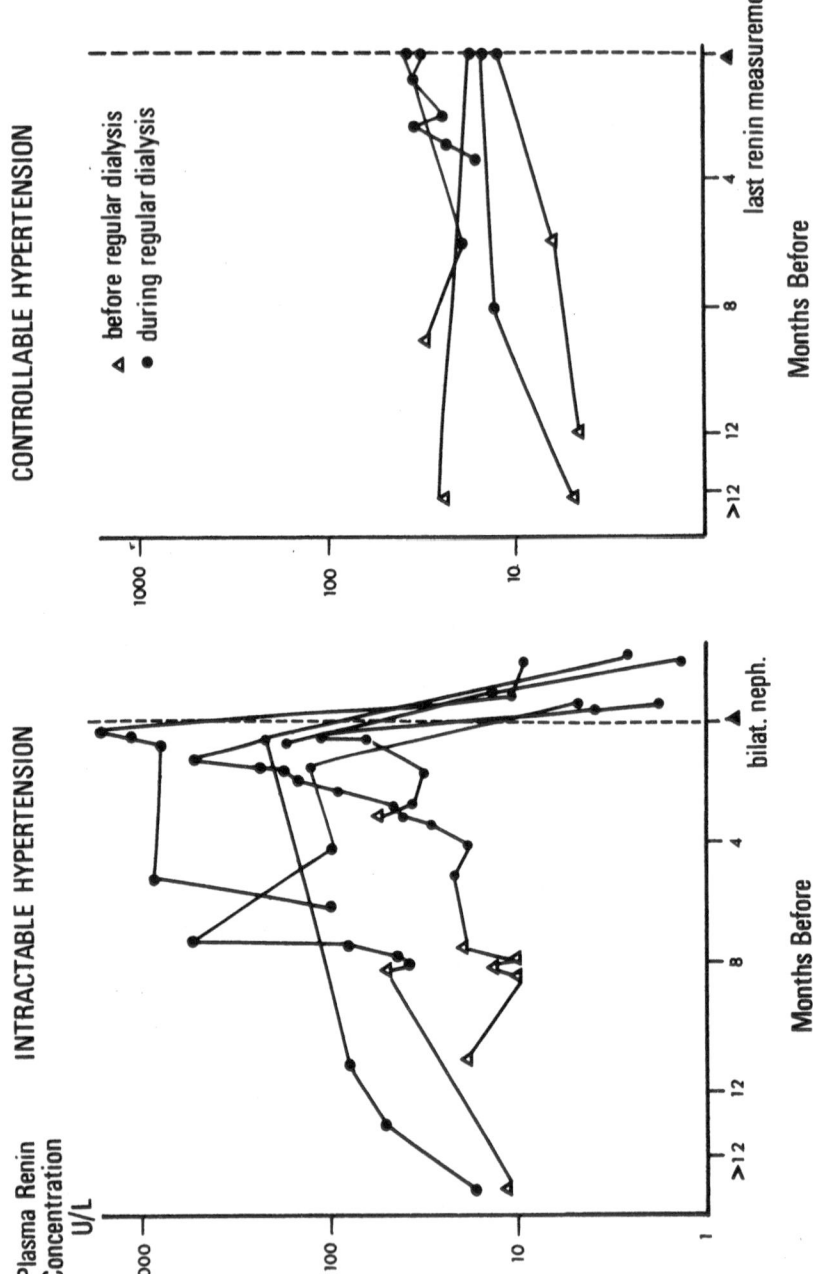

Figure 7.5 Plasma renin in chronic renal failure patients with hypertension before ($\triangle$) and during ($\bullet$) regular dialysis. On the left are five patients with intractable hypertension and on the right five patients with hypertension which was controlled by dialysis.

to sodium depletion during dialysis. Following bilateral nephrectomy there was a dramatic fall in plasma renin levels. The five patients whose blood pressure was controlled by sodium removal had plasma renin levels which were within the normal range or only slightly elevated, with no significant rise in response to sodium removal by dialysis.

Thus the hypertension found in the majority of regular dialysis patients is sodium dependent and the blood pressure can be controlled by removal of sodium and water during dialysis. In the few remaining patients, plasma renin levels are high, blood pressure cannot be controlled by sodium removal, and bilateral nephrectomy may be required.

7.2 MANAGEMENT OF HYPERTENSION

The pattern illustrated diagrammatically in Figure 7.6 is a familiar one. In patients with progressive chronic renal failure, renal function will deteriorate slowly with the passage of time. This is often associated with a

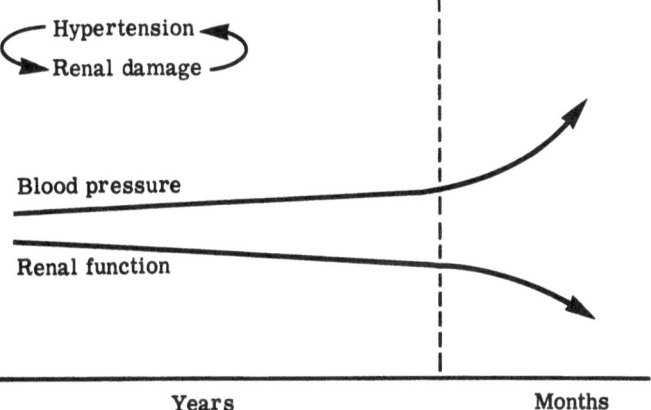

Figure 7.6 Diagrammatic representation of relationship between blood pressure and renal function in chronic renal failure

slow rise in blood pressure, but a stage may be reached when the hypertension suddenly enters an accelerated or malignant phase. This is commonly accompanied by a much more rapid decline in renal function. Thus, good blood pressure control is essential if unnecessarily rapid deterioration in renal function is to be avoided. Several drugs are available for the control of hypertension. Of those routinely available, there is no one drug or combination of drugs which has been shown to be markedly superior to the remainder. β-Adrenergic blocking drugs have been shown to inhibit the effect of renin[5] and therefore in theory should be useful in states of 'high renin' hypertension. Our experience is that while they may be effective in this situation they are by no means invariably so. Hydralazine, which has a direct relaxant effect on vascular smooth muscle, is a useful drug and is probably best used in combination with β-blockade. Thiazide diuretics, methyl dopa, clonidine and prazosin all have a place either on their own or in combination. Bethanidine is a less satisfactory drug than those just mentioned in view of the undesirable degree of postural hypotension which it often produces.

Finally minoxidil (6-imino-1,2-dihydro-1-hydroxy-2-imino-4-piperidinopyrimidine) has been shown to be a potent antihypertensive in patients with renal and other forms of hypertension[6,7]. Minoxidil has a direct relaxant effect on vascular smooth muscle and in addition has two other almost invariable effects, an increase in heart rate and sodium retention[8]. To counteract these two effects it should be given with a β-adrenergic blocking drug and with a diuretic. Forty-four patients, half of whom had impaired renal function, have been treated with minoxidil in the Glasgow

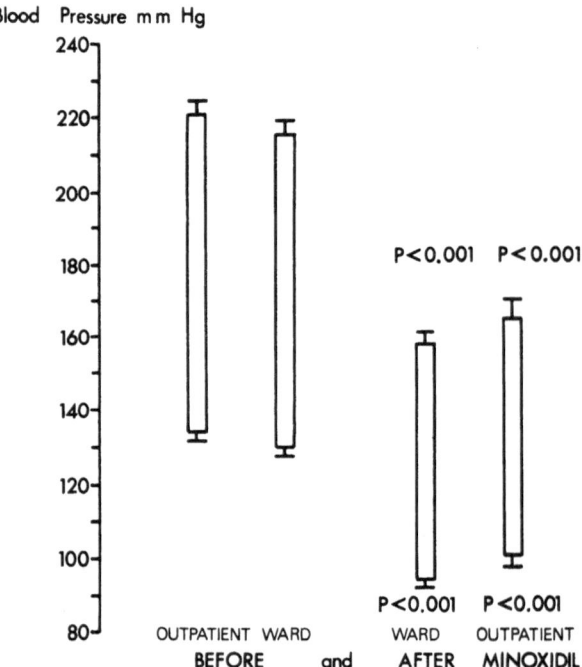

Figure 7.7 Mean supine blood pressure in 44 patients, 22 of whom had impaired renal function, before and after the administration of minoxidil

Blood Pressure Clinic. All were refractory to the commonly used anti-hypertensive drugs with diastolic blood pressure levels greater than 120 mmHg despite treatment. Figure 7.7 shows that blood pressure control with minoxidil was excellent both in the ward and later under out-patient conditions. Side-effects in these 44 patients consisted of fluid retention with left ventricular failure in three patients, gynaecomastia in three patients and invariable hirsutism. While not of undue consequence in the male, the degree of hirsutism in the female patients was disfiguring, but could be markedly improved by the use of a depilating cream.

7.3 HYPERTENSION IN PATIENTS UNDERGOING REGULAR HAEMODIALYSIS

In the majority of patients blood pressure can be controlled by removal of sodium and water during dialysis. Using changes in body weight as an index of alteration in body water and salt content, Figure 7.8 shows how

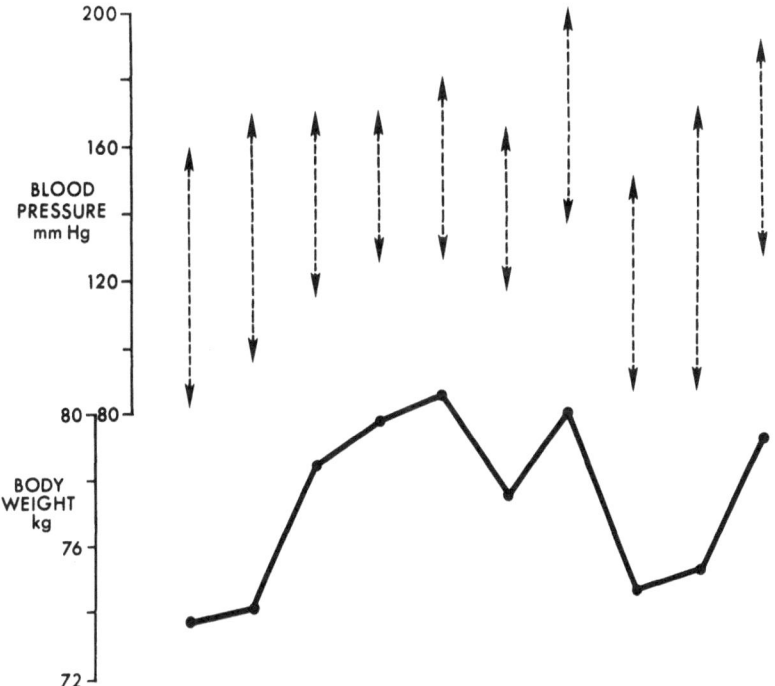

Figure 7.8   Serial supine blood pressure and body weight measurements in a regular dialysis patient showing the close relationship between blood pressure and body weight

these correlate closely with blood pressure. The proportion of patients whose blood pressure can be controlled by dialysis alone varies between centres, but the usual proportion is in the range 70–80%[9,10]. In most of the remaining patients, adequate blood-pressure control can be achieved by the use of antihypertensive drugs, but a small group of patients remain whose blood pressure is refractory to both dialysis and drugs. In the Western Infirmary, 8% of dialysis patients have been in this third group and in several cases, bilateral nephrectomy has had to be performed as an emergency because of the severity of the hypertension. Although in our experience the blood-pressure response to bilateral nephrectomy has almost always been excellent[11], there is a significant morbidity. Of the 12 patients nephrectomized in the Western Infirmary because of intractable hypertension, five developed major post-operative complications, and one of these died. A further two patients developed minor complications. In addition to the immediate post-operative morbidity, a fall in haemoglobin invariably occurred, leading to a reduced quality of health and sometimes the need for regular blood transfusion.

Because of the undesirable effects of bilateral nephrectomy, patients should be carefully assessed before the decision is taken to proceed with

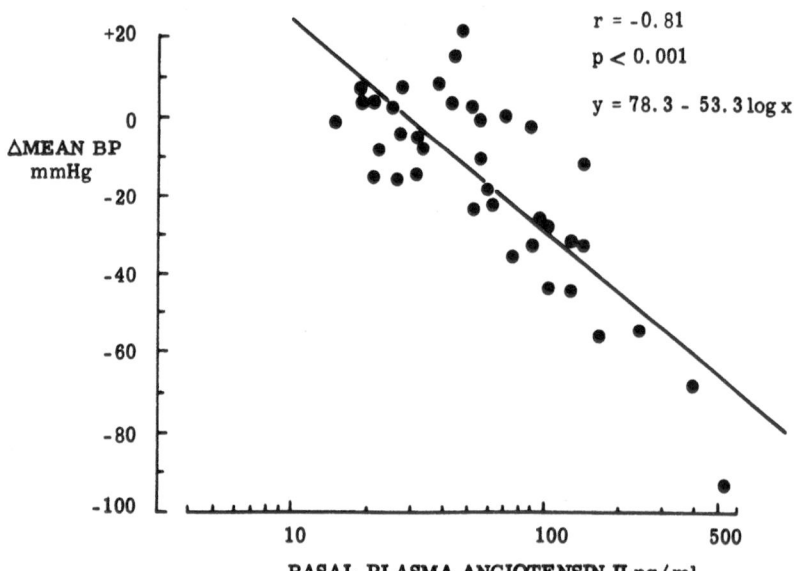

Figure 7.9   Basal plasma angiotensin II plotted against the change in mean blood pressure during the infusion of saralasin in 38 patients with various types of hypertension

this operation. Three criteria can be used. Firstly in all cases the patient should have hypertension which is refractory to dialysis and drugs. Secondly, the plasma renin or angiotensin II level should be significantly elevated or thirdly, as an alternative, the blood pressure should fall during the infusion of saralasin.

Saralasin is an octapeptide with six of its amino acid constituents identical to those of angiotensin II. Only the two terminal amino acids differ, saralasin containing sarcosine and alanine while angiotensin II contains asparagine and phenylalanine. As a consequence of its chemical similarity, saralasin acts as a competitive inhibitor to the action of angiotensin II. A saralasin infusion will therefore lower the blood pressure in patients with high plasma angiotensin II levels. Figure 7.9 shows the good

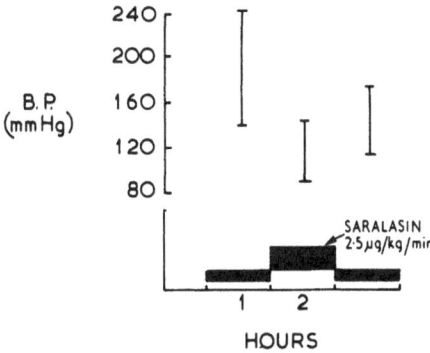

Figure 7.10   Supine blood pressure before, during and after the infusion of saralasin in a regular dialysis patient with intractable hypertension

correlation which exists between the degree of blood pressure fall during a saralasin infusion and the plasma angiotensin II levels. The figure was compiled with results from patients with a variety of types of hypertension. Most of the dialysis patients with severe hypertension are represented by circles in the bottom right-hand corner as they have much higher plasma angiotensin II levels than most other hypertensive patients. Figure 7.10 shows an example of the blood-pressure lowering effect of a saralasin infusion in a dialysis patient with intractable hypertension. This patient subsequently had an excellent blood-pressure response to bilateral nephrectomy. A saralasin infusion can therefore predict whether hypertension is likely to benefit from bilateral nephrectomy and provides useful confirmation of the significance of a high plasma angiotensin II level. It can also provide sufficient information on its own should plasma renin or angiotensin II measurements not be available.

Treatment policy in the Western Infirmary for dialysis patients with intractable hypertension is currently changing for two reasons. Firstly there is concern with regard to the morbidity associated with bilateral nephrectomy. Secondly the availability of minoxidil, with its markedly superior effect to previously available antihypertensives, has reduced the need for nephrectomy.

We have treated with minoxidil three dialysis patients whose blood pressure was resistant to dialysis and conventional antihypertensive drugs. The mean lying blood pressure on conventional drug therapy was 198/124. At 2–4 months after starting minoxidil the mean lying blood pressure had fallen to 148/89. This blood-pressure response was not associated with any side-effects nor was it due to any concomitant reduction in body weight.

7.4   BLOOD PRESSURE FOLLOWING RENAL TRANSPLANTATION

Forty-one patients were picked at random from those followed up for at least 2 years after successful transplantation. Twenty-two of these patients were on antihypertensive therapy at this time. Fourteen of the 41 patients had, for various reasons, had bilateral nephrectomy performed prior to transplantation. Only 7% of the nephrectomized patients were receiving antihypertensive therapy compared to 78% of those not previously nephrectomized. Very similar figures were reported by Cohen in a series of 81 patients[12]. Thus pre-transplant bilateral nephrectomy, irrespective of the indication for its performance, undoubtedly has a beneficial effect on blood pressure following transplantation. Curtis et al. showed that additional factors favouring a normal blood pressure were good graft function, the use of living related, as against cadaver donors, and alternate-day steroid therapy[13].

7.5   CONCLUSIONS

Blood pressure can be controlled in most regular haemodialysis patients by a combination of a low sodium intake and removal of excess sodium by dialysis. Some patients, however, require antihypertensive drugs as well. In a small number, 5–10% in most series, blood-pressure control is poor and our policy until now has been bilateral nephrectomy in these patients. In the future, the use of minoxidil will reduce though not eliminate the need for nephrectomy. Care is required to ensure that a reduction in the incidence of nephrectomy does not lead to the presence of too many severely hypertensive patients following transplantation. It could be argued that the operative morbidity of nephrectomy would be lower in transplanted compared to dialysis patients and the disadvantage of a further fall in haemoglobin would not apply. While this is probably true, it is very difficult following transplantation to determine if the elevated blood pressure is due to ischaemia of the transplant or to the patient's own kidneys. Thus there remains a definite place for pre-transplant bilateral nephrectomy in the patient with intractable hypertension although the frequency with which this operation will be performed in the future will be less than in the past.

References

1. Brown, J. J., Dusterdieck, G. O., Fraser, R., Lever, A. F., Robertson, J. I. S., Tree, M. and Weir, R. J. (1971). Hypertension and chronic renal failure. *Br. Med. Bull.*, 27, 128
2. Davies, D. L., Beevers, D. G., Brown, J. J., Fraser, R., Ferriss, J. B., Lever, A. F., Medina, A., Morton, J. J. and Robertson, J. I. S. (1973). Sodium and the renin-angiotensin system in patients with hypertension. *Proc. IVth Int. Congr. Endocrinol.*
3. Schelekamp, M. A., Beevers, D. G., Briggs, J. D., Brown, J. J., Davies, D. L., Fraser, R., Lebel, M., Lever, A. F., Medina, A., Morton, J. J., Robertson, J. I. S. and Tree, M. (1973). Hypertension in chronic renal failure: an abnormal relation between sodium and the renin–angiotensin system. *Am. J. Med.*, 55, 379
4. Brown, J. J., Curtis, J. R., Lever, A. F., Robertson, J. I. S., De Wardener, H. E. and Wing, A. J. (1969). Plasma renin concentration and the control of blood pressure in patients on maintenance haemodialysis. *Nephron*, 6, 329
5. Bühler, F. R., Laragh, J. H., Baer, L., Vaughan, E. D. and Brunner, H. R. (1972). Propranolol inhibition of renin secretion. *N. Engl. J. Med.*, 287, 1209
6. Gottlieb, T. B., Katz, F. H. and Chidsey, C. A. (1972). Combined therapy with vasodilator drugs and beta-adrenergic blockade. *Circulation*, 45, 571
7. Limas, C. J. and Freis, E. D. (1973). Minoxidil in severe hypertension with renal failure. *Am. J. Cardiol.*, 31, 355
8. Gilmore, E., Weil, J. and Chidsey, C. (1970). Treatment of essential hypertension with a new vasodilator in combination with beta-adrenergic blockade. *N. Engl. J. Med.*, 282, 521
9. Chrysanthakopoulos, S. G., Kastagir, B. K., Jubiz, W. and Kolff, W. J. (1972). Hypertension in patients on maintenance hemodialysis: evaluation of peripheral renin activity and bilateral nephrectomy. *Am. J. Med. Sci.*, 264, 9
10. Hull, A. R., Long, D. L., Prati, R. C., Pettinger, W. A. and Parker III, T. F. (1975). The control of hypertension in patients undergoing regular maintenance dialysis. *Kidney Int.*, 7, (Suppl. 2), 184
11. Medina, A., Bell, P. R. F., Briggs, J. D., Brown, J. J., Fine, A., Lever, A. F., Morton, J. J., Paton, A. M., Robertson, J. I. S., Tree, M., Waite, M. A., Weir, R. and Winchester, J. (1972). Changes of blood pressure, renin and angiotensin after bilateral nephrectomy in patients with chronic renal failure. *Br. Med. J.*, 4, 694

12.   Cohen, S. L. (1973). Hypertension in renal transplant recipients: role of bilateral nephrectomy. *Br. Med. J.*, 3, 78
13.   Curtis, J. J., Galla, J. H., Kotchen, T. A., Lucas, B., McRoberts, J. W. and Luke, R. G. (1976). Prevalence of hypertension in a renal transplant population on alternate-day steroid therapy. *Clin. Nephrol.*, 5, 123

DISCUSSION

Unidentified speaker: When groups of antihypertensives were used, did several of the patients develop postural hypotension on or off dialysis?

Briggs: It was not a major problem. We have tended recently to concentrate on β-blockers and this has not been a problem with them. It is with some of the other hypertensives. Bethanidine is obviously a good example of a drug which would never be used nowadays.

Unidentified speaker: Has there been any evidence of patients presenting with so-called 'rigid vessels', and postural dropping whilst dialysing?

Briggs: We have had no trouble with that. Our policy is slightly different from average in that our patients tend to have relatively small weight gains between dialysis. They tend to put on less weight, perhaps 1 kg or 1.5 kg between dialysis, which is less than in many centres.

Unidentified speaker: How long between dialysis?

Briggs: Thrice a week.

J. A. Kanis (Oxford): I find the interrelationships between measurements such as vascular volume, renin and blood pressure, which all seem to be interdependent, difficult to understand. I wonder whether partial correlations between them have been studied in an attempt to identify causal relationships. It is difficult to infer causal influences from correlations.

I ask this because Dr Briggs mentioned that the effects of saralasin might provide the basis for a test to decide whether a patient's hypotension might respond to bilateral nephrectomy. It seems possible that the response of any hypertensive patient might be augmented by volume depletion and that volume status should be taken into account before the saralasin effect can be interpreted.

Secondly, what is the evidence that hypertension in patients with disturbed renal function has any deleterious effect on their renal tissue?

Briggs: The first point is very valid.When a saralasin test is done it is necessary to make sure that one is not dealing with a volume-depleted or sodium-depleted patient, because that would give different results. We, as a standard, always do the saralasin test immediately prior to dialysis so that we are dealing with a relatively salt-repleted patient.

There is an anecdotal impression that hypertension does destroy renal tissue. I have seen several patients whose function has deteriorated rapidly when they have entered an accelerated hypertensive phase. I am not too well up in the literature in terms of careful and full studies but it is certainly my impression, and I think that it is a fairly general impression.

J. S. Cameron: I was interested in exactly this question in patients with glomerular disease and I hunted the literature high and low to find any evidence of whether this widespread impression was indeed true. I came up with only one paper[1], a combined university/clinic 19-centre retrospective survey from Germany published in German. Retrospective data had been analysed out in terms of blood pressure, correcting out for the type of histology with and without hypertension. Hypertension had an undoubted deleterious effect in this retrospective survey – which is one of the problems with data of that kind.

As far as I am aware it is the only evidence, and there is no other prospective study, controlled or uncontrolled.

Kanis: I bring this up because we have been looking at the rate of fall of creatinine as the reciprocal of function and we have been rather impressed to find that in some patients who have started off with normotension and who have developed hypertension, the slope has not changed when they have become quite markedly hypertensive, and has, further, not changed when that hypertension has been treated.

Briggs: Possibly there is a difference where there is severe hypertension.

R. Ahmad (Liverpool): What does Dr Briggs consider to be the optimum concentration of sodium in the dialysis solution? It amazes me that the dialysis solution supplied to NHS hospitals should vary between 120 and 145 mmol.

Briggs: It is not necessary to control hypertension by running with a low dialysate sodium.

We ourselves have not tried to run at a relatively high level. I know of experiments running at 141. We run at a sodium concentration of 137 mmol/l which seems fairly average.

Reference

1. Sarre, H. *et al*. 1971. Nephrotisches Syndrom des Erwachsenenalters. *Deutsche Med. Wochenschr.*, **96**, 225

8

Dialysis encephalopathy
M. K. Ward and
T. G. Feest

8.1 INTRODUCTION

Efficient dialysis brings about a rapid reversal of the neurological syndromes seen with 'end-stage uraemia'. Sensorial clouding, perceptual errors, hallucinations, asterixis, myoclonus, focal and grand mal seizures, decerebrate and decorticate postures are all improved by adequate haemodialysis (see Raskin and Fisherman for review)[1,2]. However patients whose lives have been prolonged by intermittent dialysis may develop other encephalopathic features. Before discussing 'dialysis encephalopathy' the differential diagnosis must be considered.

8.2 DIFFERENTIAL DIAGNOSIS

Neurological signs and symptoms are frequently seen in patients maintained on regular dialysis and have many causes. Patients may develop neurological sequelae of their primary disease process, such as hypertension or disseminated lupus erythematosis. Clouding of consciousness, delirium and hallucinations may accompany intercurrent infection, septicaemia, meningitis or encephalitis.

The metabolism and excretion of many drugs or their metabolites are altered by impaired renal function[3]. Dementia-like syndromes with or without speech disorders have been described with hypnotics, sedatives, tranquillizers, anti-parkinsonian drugs and antiepileptic therapy[4]. The benzodiazepines (flurazepam and diazepam) have been shown to produce encephalopathic syndromes[5]. Little is known about the effects of long-term administration of these drugs in dialysis patients or the possible potentiation with other drugs in uraemic man. Intermittent heparinization or continued anticoagulation exposes haemodialysis patients to the risk of subdural haematoma[6].

Because we rely on a mechanical device to maintain 'normal' levels of sodium, potassium, calcium and magnesium during dialysis there is a potential danger that acute or chronic alterations in the concentration of the dialysate due to mal-functioning proportionating units (despite so-called fail-safe devices) can lead to syndromes presenting as alteration of neurological function. Sodium and water depletion in hot weather and anaemia can present as neurological syndromes. Headache, nausea, vomiting, delirium, convulsions and obtundation are associated with fluid and electrolyte shifts produced by haemodialysis (disequilibrium syndrome)[2] and have been attributed to changes in osmotic pressure and pH within the brain and CSF[7]. Because the semi-permeable membrane is a passive device essential substances as well as 'toxins' can transfer out of or into the patient during haemodialysis. An encephalopathic syndrome attributed to thiamine deficiency has been described[8]. Acute copper intoxication has been described due to rapid transfer of copper from dialysate to blood showing that dialysate contaminated with trace elements can cause toxic symptoms[9].

8.3   DIALYSIS ENCEPHALOPATHY SYNDROME

8.3.1   Introduction

First described by Alfrey[10] in 1972 this neurological syndrome has become well documented in Europe (150 cases recorded at EDTA, Helsinki, 1977), Japan[11], Australia[12] and centres in the USA[13,14], and has been a significant cause of death in dialysis populations.

8.3.2   Clinical description of neurological syndrome (Newcastle-upon-Tyne)

Between 1970 and May 1977, 17 patients on haemodialysis were seen with this neurological syndrome. Fifteen presented with a distinctive intermittent slurring of speech towards the end of dialysis or within a few minutes of the termination of dialysis. This was often first noted by relatives or nursing staff. Two patients presented with fits 6 months before their speech disorder became apparent. Patients deteriorated over a period of 5 to 17 months to a stage where they were unable to speak or talk intelligibly. All patients developed intellectual impairment progressing in nine to global dementia and death. Disordered motor function varied from myoclonic jerks of facial muscles and limbs to widespread muscular spasms involving the whole of the body. These were often precipitated by attempted speech, lifting limbs against gravity or walking. Personality changes, depression, aggressive outbursts and emotional lability were prominent features in five of the patients. Six patients developed a cerebellar syndrome characterized by incoordination of limbs or speech associated with a fatigue phenomenon, accurate limb movements and speech becoming disorganized after a few minutes' effort which improved after a period of rest.

The most useful diagnostic test was an electroencephalogram which showed a distinctive pattern with an increase in slow wave activity associated with spike and slow wave bursts[14, 15].

We have been impressed with the close association of this syndrome and the osteomalacic type of renal ostedystrophy seen in patients on intermittent haemodialysis in the Northern Region[16]. Fifteen of the 17 patients had evidence of bone pain or myopathy and 14 out of 15 patients who had bone biopsies showed the picture commonly seen in Newcastle of osteomalacia with little or no osteitis fibrosa. Platts[17], Flendrig[18] and Alfrey[19] have also noted this association of the encephalopathic syndrome with renal osteodystrophy.

8.3.3 Therapy

No successful therapy has been reported. Attempts with levodopa, dimercaprol, penicillamine, rubidium, dexamethasone, physostigmine, vitamins[11] and bromocryptine[40] have all failed. Myoclonic jerks and grand mal seizures can be controlled with intermittent diazepam or clonazepam. Three of our patients remained static with little progression of encephalopathy over 3–9 months when phosphate binders were discontinued and they were transferred to a deionized water supply. Improvement has been seen in two patients who had successful renal transplantation[20], although five other patients reported from the same unit showed progressive deterioration after renal transplantation despite good renal function. This experience of the failure of transplantation to affect the progression of the neurological disease is the more commonly reported outcome[16, 17]. In fact, Platts[17] reported the presentation of the syndrome following successful renal transplantation. Improvement has been reported in one case following parathyroidectomy and hypercalcaemia was thought to be a contributing factor only[21].

8.3.4 Histopathology

No gross macroscopic abnormalities in the brain have been reported. The documented abnormalities were histopathological. Features noted included astrocyte proliferation with neuronal loss in the cortex, and purkinge cell loss with Bergman gliosis in the cerebellum[11, 16]. This lack of specific histological and macroscopic abnormalities suggest that the aetiology is probably a toxic metabolic encephalopathy[11].

8.4 AETIOLOGY OF DIALYSIS ENCEPHALOPATHY

8.4.1 Introduction

There are no histological features that suggest either known bacteriological or virus infection as the aetiological agent. A 'slow' virus is an alternative hypothesis but to date no animal passage experiments performed either in the USA or in the UK have reproduced the encephalopathic syndrome.

Maintenance haemodialysis exposes patients to the risk of a 'deficiency syndrome' or the accumulation of a 'toxic substance'. It seems unlikely that the distinct geographical distribution of this syndrome can be accounted for by minor differences in dialysis technique, or by a deficiency syndrome produced by dialysis. It seems more likely that the distinct geographical distribution supports the hypothesis that it is an accumulation of one or more toxic substances.

8.4.2   Evidence for aluminium as the possible 'toxin'

Aluminium is the most plentiful metal in the earth's crust and is only exceeded in abundance by silica and oxygen. Unlike other metals no biological functions have been demonstrated for aluminium and there is no evidence that it is a major coenzyme factor in man[22]. Although exposure of man to aluminium is inevitable there are very few reports of illness in workers working in the production and processing of aluminium which has been directly attributed to aluminium toxicity. The commonest problem encountered is that of pulmonary fibrosis in workers exposed to pulverised aluminium metal[23]. However McLaughlin and co-workers[24] described one man working in a ball mill using aluminium flake powder who developed a strikingly similar encephalopathic syndrome to that described in our dialysis patients. Tissue aluminium levels in this patient were found to be extremely high.

A recent review of studies in laboratory animals with orally administered aluminium compounds documents the conflicting results obtained[22]. It appears that if hypophosphataemia is avoided then there is little evidence of aluminium being toxic when given orally, although there is inconclusive evidence that aluminium-loaded animals may have a disturbance of phosphate metabolism even when hypophosphataemia is avoided[25].

However, the direct application of aluminium-containing compounds to nervous tissue in animal models was first shown to be toxic more than 30 years ago[26].

8.4.3   Accumulation of aluminium in man

The total body burden of aluminium may be increased by absorption from the gastrintestinal tract or by direct parenteral administration. Clarkson and colleagues[27] performed balanced studies on patients with chronic renal failure receiving aluminium-containing phosphate binders which showed that they could easily be placed in a positive aluminium balance. Kaehny and colleagues[28] showed a rise in plasma aluminium levels and urinary excretion of aluminium in normal subjects taking aluminium-containing compounds. A recent survey[29] showed that ingestion of aluminium-containing compounds among haemodialysis patients in Europe did not correlate with the encephalopathic syndrome. If aluminium accumulation is the cause of dementia this suggests that the gastrointestinal tract may not be the major source of aluminium in patients maintained on intermittent haemodialysis or the prescribed dose was not ingested by the patients. However, we have seen one patient with chronic renal failue not on intermittent haemodialysis who was given aluminium hydroxide 80–100 ml daily for 12 months and regular monthly estimations of serum phosphate showed that she never became hypophosphataemic. This patient developed myopathy, bone pain and dementia. Histopathology showed that her bone lesion was predominantly osteomalacia with little osteitis fibrosa, a similar picture to that seen in patients on haemodialysis in Newcastle-upon-Tyne[30].

The major source of aluminium appears to be the water supply used in the preparation of dialysate for haemodialysis. Flendrig, Krus and Das[18] reported the appearance of the encephalopathic syndrome associated with myopathy and fractured bones in patients dialysed in his unit which used the same water supply as another unit where the syndrome was not seen. It was found that aluminium electrodes placed in the water supply to his dialysis unit had dissolved and that the water supply had become contaminated with aluminium. The other dialysis unit had not used the same aluminium electrode system. There was a striking increase in the tissue level of aluminium in the patients dying of encephalopathy in his dialysis unit compared to patients dying with normal renal function, patients dying with chronic renal failure and patients with chronic renal failure who were dialysed in other centres in Holland.

This is the nearest to a double-blind control trial of intravenously administered aluminium compounds that is ever likely to be carried out in man. Previously, Alfrey and associates[31] had studied a considerable number of trace metals in the tissues of patients dying of chronic uraemia and dialysis encephalopathy (Cu, Fe, Zn, As, Se, Br, Rb, Si, Mo, Cd, Sn, Pb and Al). They found a strikingly significant elevation in the aluminium content of the tissues of patients dying with encephalopathy when compared with patients dying with normal renal function and dialysis patients dying of other causes. Table 8.1 documents the tissue aluminium content of dialysed uraemic patients who died of other causes (DO) compared to those who died with encephalopathy (DE) and a control group who died

TABLE 8.1 Tissue aluminium in dialysed uraemic patients who died of other causes (DO) compared to those who died with encephalopathy (DE) and a control group who died with normal renal function (C)

Author	Method	C	DO	DE
(A) Brain (mg/kg)				
Flendrig 1976[18]	NA	11.9 (2)*	12.1 (2)	90.8 (4)
Alfrey 1976[19]	FAAS	1.3 (6)†	7.63 (6)	24.98 (6) (grey matter)
Ward 1976[16]	FAAS	9.5 (4)†	—	26.5 (4) (grey matter)
(B) Liver (mg/kg)				
Flendrig 1976[18]	NA	15.8 (7)*	32.9 (5)	610.2 (4)
Alfrey 1976[19]	FAAS	4.3 (11)†	182.0 (6)	381.0 (14)
(C) Bone (mg/kg)				
Flendrig 1976[18]	NA	10.6 (4)*	23.5 (5)	272.0 (2)
Alfrey 1976[19]	FAAS	2.4 (7)†	104.0 (28)	251.0 (12)

NA = Neutron activation
FAAS = Flameless atomic absorption spectrophotometry
* Dry tissue
† Dry defatted tissue
( ) = Numer of studies

with normal renal function (C). It has been known since 1971[32] that patients in Newcastle have had a high aluminium content in their bones, and in four patients with dialysis encephalopathy frontal lobe grey matter had elevated aluminium levels when compared with a control group[16]. Four dialysis units in the United Kingdom account for 70% of the case reports of patients with the encephalopathic syndrome (Plymouth, Leeds, Sheffield, Newcastle)[33]. In all these areas there is either naturally high aluminium content in the water or alum precipitation is used as a method of water treatment (range of aluminium level is 30–1200 μg/l)[34]. Among 12 renal units in the London area dialysis encephalopathy is rare and 'Newcastle bone disease' uncommon. The water supply to the renal units in London is from supplies that do not normally use alum coagulation and do not have a high natural aluminium content to the water (aluminium level usually less than 50 μg/l)[34].

Aluminium is not removed efficiently by water softeners or by a weak based deionizer which is nearing regeneration. Aluminium appears to be most efficiently removed by reverse osmosis with or without polishing deionization depending on the reverse osmosis unit used providing the unit and membrane are intact[35].

8.5   PREVENTION BY ADEQUATE WATER TREATMENT

The failure to treat effectively the encephalopathic syndrome and the osteo-malacic type of bone disease suggests that the metabolic inhibitor or inhibitors causes irreversible alteration to the metabolic mechanisms effected or is so well bound within the body that it is not easily removed. It has been shown[36-38] that prevention by adequate water treatment from the initiation of haemodialysis is the most effective treatment for severe osteomalacic bone disease. No patients treated for the whole of their dialysis history on deionized water in Newcastle have developed encephalopathy.

The correlation of tissue aluminium content with duration of dialysis[19] may suggest that the accumulation is passive and the metal inert. Cartier[39] found high tissue levels in dialysed patients with or without the encephalopathic syndrome. The dose and rate of aluminium accumulation and individual patient differences to increased total body aluminium have not been studied in man. It is possible that aluminium needs another factor or is a marker and these water supplies have an unassociated but as yet undetermined toxin.

8.6   CONCLUSIONS

1. Neurological syndromes presenting in patients on haemodialysis are not uncommon and may be due to a variety of factors.
2. Dialysis encephalopathy syndrome is a distinct neurological syndrome, usually associated with myopathy and bone disease, characterized by osteomalacia with little or no osteitis fibrosa.
3. Higher tissue aluminium levels have been demonstrated in patients dying with the dialysis encephalopathy syndrome than dialysis patients dying of other causes in Europe, Australia and the USA.
4. The geographical distribution of the encephalopathic syndrome within the UK is associated with areas known to have a high natural aluminim content of the water or where alum precipitation is used in the water treatment.
5. Aluminium is not removed efficiently by water softeners, the most commonly used water treatment for haemodialysis in the UK.
6. The above evidence is highly suggestive that aluminium is toxic to uraemic man maintained on intermittent haemodialysis though the mechanism is not understood.
7. Adequate water treatment from the initiation of dialysis appears to prevent the development of dialysis encephalopathy and the associated osteomalacic type of renal osteodystrophy.

ACKNOWLEDGEMENTS

We are indebted to Professor D. N. S. Kerr for unending help and encouragement, to Professor D. A. S. Shaw and members of the Department of Neurology, Professor B. Tomlinson and Dr R. Perry of the Department of Neuropathology and the Scientific Services of the Regional Water Authorities for providing data on the aluminium content of the water supplies.

References

1. Raskin, M. M. and Fishman, A. R. (1976). Neurological disorders in renal failure (Part I). *N. Engl. J. Med.*, **294**, 3, 143
2. Raskin, M. M. and Fishman, A. R. (1976). Neurological disorders in renal failure (Part II). *N. Engl. J. Med.*, **294**
3. Kerr, D. N. S., Dettli, L., Rawlins, M., Leber, H. W. and Maddocks, J. (1976). Drug metabolism in uraemic renal failure. *Proc. ED.T.A.*, **13**, 597 (London: Pitman Medical)
4. McCelland, M. A. (1977). Psychiatric Disorders. In O. M. Davis (ed.). *Textbook of Adverse Drug Reactions*, pp. 335–349 (Oxford: Oxford University Press)
5. Taclob, L. and Needle, M. (1976). Drug induced encephalopathy in patients on maintenance haemodialysis. *Lancet*, **ii**, 704
6. Leonard, A. and Shapiro, F. L. (1975). Subdural haematoma in regularly haemodialysed patients. *Ann. Intern. Med.*, **82**, 650
7. Arieff, A. Z., Massiz, S. G. and Bonientos, A. (1973). Brain water and electrolyte metabolism in uraemia, effects of slow and rapid haemodialysis. *Kidney Int.*, **4**, 177
8. Lopez, R. I. and Collins, G. K. (1968). Wernicke's encephalopathy: a complication of chronic haemodialysis. *Arch. Neurol.*, **18**, 248
9. Lyle, H. I., Payton, J. E. and Hui, M. (1976). Haemodialysis and copper fever. *Lancet*, **i**, 1324
10. Alfrey, A. C., Mischell, J. M., Barks, J. S., Coniguglia, S. R., Rudolph, M., Lewine E. and Holmes, J. M. (1977). Syndrome of praxia and multifocal seizures associated with haemodialysis. *Trans. Am. Soc. Artif. Intern. Organs*, **18**, 257
11. Barks, J. S., Alfrey, A. C., Huddlestone, J., Norenberg, M. D. and Lewine, E. (1976). A fatal encephalopathy in chronic haemdialysis patients, *Lancet*, **ii**, 764
12. Barratt, L. J. and Lawrence, J. R. (1975). Dialysis associated dementia. *Aust. N. Z. J. Med.*, **5**, 62
13. Mahurkar, S. D., Dhar, S. R., Saltra, R., Meyers, L., Smith, E. C. and Dunea, G. (1973). Dialysis dementia, *Lancet*, **1**, 1412
14. Chokroverty, S., Bruetman, M. E., Berger, V. and Reyes, M. G. (1976). Progressive dialytic encephalopathy. *J. Neurol., Neurosurg. Psychiat.*, **39**, 411
15. Nodel, A. M., Wilson, W. P. (1976). Dialysis encephalopathy: a possible seizure disorder. *Neurology*, **26**, 1130

16. Ward, M. K., Pierides, A. M., Fawcett, P., Shaw, D. A., Perry, A. M., Tomlinson, B. E. and Kerr, D. N. S. (1976). Dialysis encephalopathy syndrome. *Proc. E.D.T.A.*, 13, 348 (London: Pitman Medical)

17. Platts, M. M., Moorehead, P. J. and Greech (1973). Dialysis dementia. *Lancet*, ii, 159

18. Flendrig, J. A., Krus, H. and Das, H. A. (1976). Aluminium intoxication: the cause of dialysis dementia? *Proc. E.D.T.A.*, 13, 355 (London: Pitman Medical)

19. Alfrey, A. C., Le Grendrere, G. R. and Kaehny, W. P. (1976). The dialysis encephalopathy syndrome. *N. Engl. J. Med.*, 294, 184

20. Silke, B., Fitzgerald, G. R., Hanson, S., Carmody, M. and O'Dwyer, W. F. (1977). Treatment of dialysis dementia by renal transplantation, Abstract *E.D.T.A.*, Helsinki, p. 266

21. Ball, J. M., Barkas, D. E. and Madison, D. S. (1977). Effect of subtotal parathyroidectomy on dialysis dementia. *Nephron*, 18, 151

22. Sorenson, J. R. J., Campbell, R. I., Tepper, L. B. and Limgg, R. D. (1974). Aluminium in the environment and human health. *Environ. Hlth Perspect.*, 8, 3

23. Jordan, J. W. (1961). Pulmonary fibrosis in a worker using aluminium powder, *Br. J. Indust. Med.*, 18, 21.

24. McLaughlin, A. F. G., Kazantizis, G., King, E., Teare, D., Porter, R. J. and Owen, R. (1962). Pulmonary fibrosis and encephalopathy associated with inhalation of aluminium dust. *Br. J. Indust. Med.*, 19, 253

25. Ondreicka, R., Kortus, J. and Ginter, E. (1971). Aluminium: its absorption, distribution and effects on phosphorous metabolism. In S. C. Skorgra and D. Waldron-Edward (eds.). *Intestinal Absorption of Metal Ions, Trace Elements and Radio Nuclides*, p. 293 (Oxford: Pergamon Press)

26. Faeth, W. M. (1955). Threshold studies on production of experimental epilepsy with alumina cream. *Proc. Soc. Exp. Biol. Med.*, 88, 329

27. Clarkson, E. M., Lucks, V. A., Hynson, W. V., Bailey, R. R., Eastwood, J. B., Woodhead, J. S., Clements, V. R., O'Riordan, L. H. and De Warden, H. E. (1972). The effect of aluminium hydroxide on calcium, phosphorous and aluminium balances, the serum parathyroid hormone concentration and the aluminium content of bone in patients with chronic renal failure. *Clin. Sci.*, 43, 519

28. Kaehny, W. D., Hegg, A. P. and Alfrey, A. C. (1977). Gastrointestinal absorption of aluminium from aluminium containing antacids. *N. Engl. J. Med.*, 296, 1389

29. Jacobs, C., Brunner, F. P., Chantler, C., Donckerwolcke, R. A., Gurland, H. J., Hathway, R. A., Selwood, N. H. and Wing, A. J. (1977). Combined report on intermittent dialysis and renal transplantation in Europe, VII, 1976. *Proc. E.D.T.A.*, 14, 3. (London: Pitman)

30. Ellis, H. A. and Peart, K. M. (1973). Azotaemia renal osteodystrophy: a quantitative study on iliac bone. *J. Clin. Pathol.*, 26, 83

31. Alfrey, A. C., Smythe, W. R., Ibels, I. S. and Mannelly, L. L. (1976). Trace element abnormalities in chronic uraemia. *Second Annual Progress Report* (University of Colorado)

32. Parsons, V., Davis, C., Goode, C., Ogg, C. and Siddiqui, J. (1971). The aluminium content of bone in patients on haemodialysis. *Br. Med. J.*, 4, 273

33. Ward, M. K. (1977). Survey of United Kingdom Dialysis Units. (In preparation)
34. Scientific Services of the United Kingdom Water Authorities
35. Strong, A., Ward, M. K., Parkinson, I. and the Scientific Services (Wear Division), Northumbria Water Authority. (In preparation)
36. Posen, G. A., Gray, D. G., Jaworsky, R., Couture, R. and Rashid, A. (1972). Comparison of renal osteodystrophy in patients dialysed with deionised and non-deionised water. *Trans. Am. Soc. Artif. Intern. Organs.*, **18**, 405
37. Leather, H. (1975). Dialysis bone disease in Plymouth. Presented at *Dialysis Symposium 1975* (Elga Publication)
38. Kerr, D. N. S. (1977). Renal osteodystrophy (The Osmond Lecture). Presented at the Renal Association
39. Cartier, F., Allain, P., Peckers, G. J. and Garre, M. (1977). Comparative study of patients with and without encephalopathy syndrome, Abstract *E.D.T.A.*, Helsinki, p. 186
40. Ward, M. K. (1976). Unpublished observation

DISCUSSION

B. Silke (Dublin): In the 3-year period 1972–75 we had 15 cases of dialysis dementia, but unlike the Newcastle group we have had no evidence whatsoever of mineral bone disease occurring in association with this syndrome. Perhaps this reflects a local bone problem in Newcastle. None of our patients had significant osteomalacia or hypophosphataemia.

In our experience transplantation proved the only effective treatment and two patients showed significant improvement as evidenced by a reversal of clinical and EEG parameters.

However, what is important is that in an 18-month period we have seen no new cases, despite no alterations in treatment or dialysis technique. We are therefore doubtful of the aluminium intoxication theory or the significance of the various phosphate binders. We believe that this is a disease that came, and is perhaps on the wane. We are happy to see it go away because we were not able to do anything that had any effect on it. Could this syndrome be getting less, or is it just a localized phenomenon?

Ward: I do not think that it is getting less in the UK. A survey is in progress to discover whether there have been any new cases since the regional survey was completed in 1975.

At least half of our patients were on home dialysis. They used different dialysers and different types of proportionating units and we do not think that the dialyser makes any difference.

Aluminium intoxication has not been excluded. Unless the aluminium content of the water supply and the patient is known it is not possible to prove that it is not due to aluminium intoxication. We were fooled by this for a while. In fact, the aluminium in the water supply goes up and down like a yo-yo, and it can be anything from 50 μg to 1.5 mg/l in the same water supply over a period of time, and without following it regularly one can have no idea of the cumulative mean aluminium content that these patients are exposed to. Dr Silke did not say whether they measured the aluminium content in the water supply, or in the brain. I am glad to hear of the success with transplantation and that this syndrome is apparently on the wane.

We have some evidence that the aluminium content in one geographical area in the UK appeared to be satisfactory for 9 months to a year, and suddenly mean levels rose towards the end of 1976. If the experiments in animals can be extrapolated to man, then there is a delay period between the accumulation of aluminium and the clinical syndrome. Cases of dementia may be seen within the next 6–9 months. Animal experiments have shown that there is a delay before the syndrome develops once the aluminium has been given to the animals.

I do not know why aluminium is toxic. In Newcastle we are convinced that it is something in the water, and we have been suspicious of this for about 8 years. We compared ourselves with East Birmingham to see whether there was any connection with fluoride, and were unable to find any (both Newcastle and East Birmingham have fluoridated water). East Birmingham has no bone disease, and no dementia – and nor is it on an aluminium containing water supply! The aluminium-containing water supply areas are Plymouth, where there are cases of dementia and bone disease; the Leeds area, where cases of dementia and bone disease occur; Sheffield, where there are cases of dementia and bone disease, and Glasgow. I am not so sure about Glasgow. The water supply has a small amount of aluminium in it, but most of the cases in Glasgow come from the Highlands, and we hope to be able to measure the content of aluminium in the Highland water.

In the non-alum water treatment areas, London and the Thames Basin, where aluminium coagulation is not used for water treatment, there is virtually no histological Newcastle bone disease, and no dementia. Therefore the evidence epidemiologically is extremely strong.

J. A. Kanis (Oxford): That there is no clinical evidence of osteomalacia would not necessarily mean that there is no histological evidence of osteomalacia. I have certainly been impressed by the association of dialysis dementia with the histological appearance of osteomalacia. There is no proof that aluminium and dialysis dementia are causally related and the aluminium may be a marker for another compound.

Ward: I accept that, though it is difficult to interpret Dr Flendrig's data unless there is more than one toxin.

Kanis: In view of Dr Ward's comments on the possible effects of calcium phosphate transport this may be meaningful.

I read an interesting abstract – I cannot remember where – on the effects of parathyroidectomy on dialysis dementia. Would Dr Ward comment on that?

Ward: That patient was extremely hypercalcaemic, and this may have been contributing to the syndrome, but I cannot interpret that completely.

R. Ahmad (Liverpool): We must be sure to classify dementia into two categories, reversible dementia and irreversible dementia. We must be sure that we are not removing something from the patients. The artificial kidney does not perform like a normal kidney. It may be that for patients on a restricted protein diet something essential is being removed and that that, and not the aluminium, is the cause of the problem.

Ward: I entirely agree that we do not know what we are removing from our patients. We have tried to exclude the phosphate problem. We know that thiamine can cause a dementia-like syndrome. Earlier in the Paper I outlined some of the things that must be excluded – thiamine and other problems and drugs. The 'removal theory' does not explain the geographical distribution. We are now so convinced that it is a water-born toxin that we have decreed that no patient may go home unless he is on a de-ionizer, or on some form of water therapy that will remove whatever is in the water supply. I agree that aluminium may still be a marker and could accumulate in the brain as a secondary phenomenon, but I would subscribe to the view that the more likely explanation is that which I have already given, that somehow the aluminium is the toxic agent, or its metabolic influence on uraemic man is the toxic influence.

If patients continue to be dialysed on aluminium-containing water supplies I would be very interested, because in 2 or 3 years' time we would be able to compare the Newcastle group with that group and see whether we have solved the problems and they have not.

9

Anaemia in patients with chronic renal failure treated by intermittent haemodialysis – aetiology and treatment
R. J. Winney and J. S. Robson

9.1   INTRODUCTION

In recent years understanding of the pathogenesis of the anaemia associated with chronic renal failure has increased more slowly than knowledge of bone disease. As a result progress in the treatment of anaemia has been overshadowed by the more dramatic success of the synthetic vitamin D metabolites in the treatment of renal osteodystrophy. Nevertheless progress has been made and anaemia should not now severely restrict the activities of the majority of haemodialysis patients.

9.2   PATHOGENESIS OF ANAEMIA IN CHRONIC RENAL FAILURE[1-3]

The two main factors responsible for the anaemia of chronic renal failure are haemolysis and impaired erythropoiesis. The reduction in red blood cell survival correlates with the degree of uraemia[4] and results from a toxic effect of uraemia, although the mechanism is not clear. However, since the degree of haemolysis should be easily compensated for by a normally functioning marrow depressed erythropoiesis limiting production of red blood cells is probably the main mechanism[5]. Until recently the decreased erythropoiesis was believed to be due to an inhibitory effect of uraemia on bone marrow but, although the severity of anaemia parallels the degree of uraemia, this relationship varies widely from patient to patient[6]. It is now recognized that insufficient production of erythropoietin is an important, and possibly the main factor resulting in depressed erythropoiesis in chronic renal failure. Table 9.1 summarizes current knowledge concerning this hormone. The importance of erythropoietin deficiency in the patho-

TABLE 9.1   Erythropoietin – summary of current knowledge

---

1. Erythropoietin is a glycoprotein of M.W. 46 000

2. *Sites of production*
    (*a*) renal – *either* kidney synthesizes erythropoietin
                – *or* kidney synthesizes an enzyme, erythrogen, which reacts with a
                    plasma-borne substrate, produced in the liver, to generate bio-
                    logically active erythropoietin
    (*b*) extrarenal – ? liver, ? spleen

3. *Control of production* – mediated by oxygen supply relative to rate of oxygen
    consumption

4. *Substances known to stimulate erythropoietin production:*
    – androgens
    – cobalt chloride

---

genesis of renal anaemia is supported by the finding of low plasma levels
of erythropoietin in these patients compared to high levels in anaemic
patients without renal disease[7]. However, it is likely that the diseased
kidney does have some residual erythropoietin secretion since anephric
patients on haemodialysis are more severely anaemic than patients on
haemodialysis with kidneys *in situ*[8]. While the low plasma levels of erythropoietin in patients with chronic renal failure are likely to result mainly from
destruction of renal tissue, an erythropoietin inhibitory effect of uraemic
plasma has also been reported[9]. The evidence to date points to erythropoietin deficiency as the main reason for depressed erythropoiesis in
chronic renal failure. That uraemia is also a factor in the depressed erythropoiesis is suggested by the observations that a uraemic environment has an
inhibitory effect on marrow cultures[10] and that erythropoiesis improves in
haemodialysis patients without any rise in plasma erythropoietin[11].

The therapeutic role of erythropoietin in renal anaemia must await
further developments in the assay and purification of this hormone. However, a number of substances have been shown to influence erythropoietin
secretion and they might have important therapeutic implications in
patients with chronic renal failure; two such substances, androgens[12] and
cobalt chloride[13], are referred to in Sections 9.6 and 9.7.

9.3 EFFECT OF HAEMODIALYSIS ON PATHOGENETIC MECHANISMS

With regular haemodialysis haemolysis may improve slightly[1] but red
blood cell survival does not return to normal[11]. Some improvement in

erythropoiesis also occurs resulting in a tendency for the anaemia to improve slowly[6, 11], the degree of improvement being related to frequency and duration of haemodialysis[1]. The observation that the improvement in erythropoiesis occurs without any rise in plasma erythropoietin suggests that it results from improved control of uraemia[11, 14]. However, improved nutrition from an increase in protein intake may also be a factor improving erythropoiesis in haemodialysis patients[15]. Figure 9.1 shows that in our

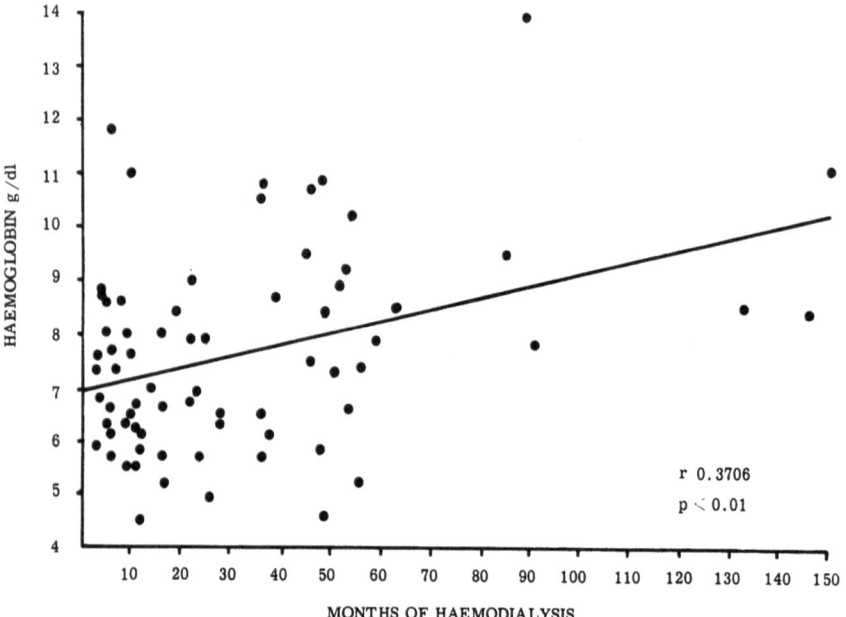

Figure 9.1 Relationship of haemoglobin to duration of haemodialysis in patients on haemodialysis

haemodialysis patients there is a tendency for the haemoglobin to rise very slowly with increasing duration of haemodialysis but there is a marked variation in the degree of anaemia at any one time. There was also no relationship in these patients between the degree of anaemia and the plasma creatinine concentration. Thus it seems likely that variation in residual erythropoietin secretion or other factors have an important role in determining the degree of anaemia in haemodialysis patients.

Although haemodialysis may lead to some improvement in anaemia, in other ways it can aggravate the anaemia, and potential improvement may thus be masked.

Chloramines, a substance used for drinking water purification all over the world, may further reduce red cell survival in patients treated by haemodialysis. Return to normal red blood cell survival has been reported using chloramine-free dialysate[16]. In addition, in some areas with a particularly high chloramine content in tap water, a significant improvement in anaemia has been described following the addition of ascorbic acid, a reducing agent, to the dialysis fluid[17].

Haemodialysis may also adversely affect erythropoiesis in two ways. Firstly, water-soluble vitamins are lost in the dialysis fluid and the loss of folic acid in particular may lead to megaloblastic erythropoiesis[18]. The regular administration of oral supplements of water-soluble vitamins prevents this potential complication. Secondly, and probably most important, haemodialysis by its very nature is associated with chronic blood loss[19-21]. Table 9.2 lists the most important reasons for this blood loss. With advances in technology blood loss during haemodialysis has been considerably reduced but a patient on regular haemodialysis treatment still loses a minimum of 3 l annually (Table 9.2). This represents a daily loss of 2 mg of

TABLE 9.2   Annual blood loss in haemodialysis patients

	Hospital dialysis twice weekly	Home dialysis thrice weekly
Blood sampling	1150 ml	300 ml
Cannulation of fistula	728 ml	1092 ml
Residual loss in dialyser	1040 ml	1560 ml
Total	2918 ml	2952 ml

iron assuming a haemoglobin of 7 g/dl and is likely to be more than this in some patients. With accurate measurements an iron loss of 5–6 mg of iron has been estimated[1]. Haemodialysis patients may therefore develop iron deficiency unless they are given iron supplements. Thus whereas iron deficiency is a minor factor in the anaemia of chronic renal failure it might become an important factor further impairing erythropoiesis in patients treated by haemodialysis.

9.4   IRON DEFICIENCY IN HAEMODIALYSIS PATIENTS

9.4.1   Incidence

In the early days of haemodialysis blood transfusion was given regularly to treat the anaemia of patients on haemodialysis. This more than compensated for blood loss and there was a real risk of iron overload[22]. However, since the risk of contracting hepatitis has been recognized blood

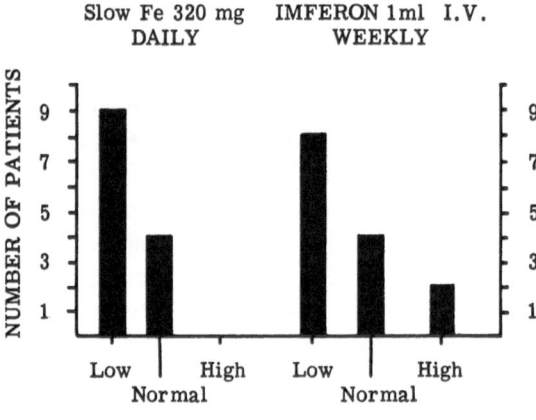

Figure 9.2   Marrow iron stores in patients on haemodialysis before treatment with oral and intravenous iron

transfusion has been restricted and many studies now reveal a high incidence of depleted iron stores in haemodialysis patients who are not taking iron supplements[23, 24]. Figure 9.2 shows the sternal marrow iron stores in two groups of patients in Edinburgh before treatment with either oral or intravenous iron. In all patients blood transfusion was used only if there was severe symptomatic anaemia or to replace major acute blood loss. Most of the patients had depleted marrow iron stores although 25% of patients had normal iron stores while in a minority the stores were high; these findings confirm previous observations. Although in the majority of patients whom we studied the plasma iron was below normal and the percentage saturation of the total iron binding capacity was low, there was a very poor correlation between both of these measurements and marrow iron stores, an observation made previously[25, 26]. Thus neither plasma iron nor percentage saturation is a reliable guide to the state of iron stores or to the need for iron supplements. Serum ferritin levels, however, correlate well with marrow iron stores in haemodialysis patients[27]. Since the measurement of serum ferritin is less disturbing to the patient than assessment of marrow iron stores it is likely to become a useful means of monitoring iron stores in haemodialysis patients.

9.4.2   Effect of iron therapy on anaemia in haemodialysis patients

Figure 9.3 shows the effect of oral and intravenous iron supplements on the haemoglobin in patients on haemodialysis. The marrow iron stores in

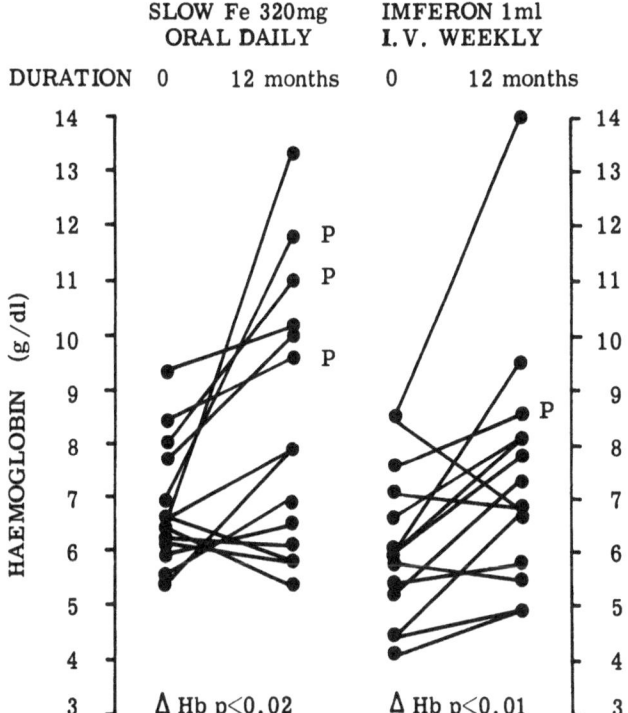

Figure 9.3 Haemoglobin before and after treatment with oral and intravenous iron in patients on haemodialysis. Values of haemoglobin for each patient before and after treatment with iron are indicated by closed circles, the two values being joined by a line. The significance of the change in haemoglobin with iron is shown for each group. P indicates patients with polycystic kidney disease

these patients before iron theapy are shown in Figure 9.2. In the majority of patients iron was given for 12 months before reassessment but some patients were reassessed earlier if other aspects of treatment altered. The patients were all treated by haemodialysis for 8 h twice weekly and were randomly allocated to one of the two treatment groups, there being 14 patients in each group. Details of these patients are shown in Table 9.3. The majority of patients were established on haemodialysis before this study but three of the patients given oral iron and one of the patients given intravenous iron commenced haemodialysis at the onset of the study. The dietary protein in all patients was 70 g daily providing 12–20 mg of elemental iron and all patients took oral supplements of a vitamin B complex tablet, ascorbic acid and folic acid. The oral iron was given as a slow release oral iron preparation (Slow Fe), in a dose of 320 mg daily before breakfast providing 100 mg of elemental iron daily. The intravenous iron was given as Imferon, 1 ml weekly providing 50 mg of elemental iron; the Imferon being given during dialysis through the venous chamber of the venous return line from the dialyser. The haemoglobin in the two groups

TABLE 9.3   Details of haemodialysis patients treated with oral and intravenous iron supplements

Treatment	Number of patients	Age (years) mean ± SEM	Duration haemodialysis (months) mean ± SEM
Slow Fe 320 mg daily (100 mg Fe)	14 (9M, 5F)	35 ± 2.9	10.5 ± 7.1
Imferon 1 ml i.v. weekly (50 mg Fe)	14 (11M, 3F)	39 ± 3.3	23.5 ± 7.4

did not differ significantly before treatment. After treatment a significant rise in haemoglobin had occurred in both groups and there was no significant difference between the response in the two groups. In individual patients however, the response was variable. In four patients given oral iron, one of whom required blood transfusion during the period of study, and in three given intravenous iron there was no rise in haemoglobin. In addition two patients given intravenous iron, in whom there was a negligible rise in haemoglobin with iron, required blood transfusion for symptomatic anaemia. At the other extreme one patient in each group, neither of whom had polycystic kidney disease, attained a normal haemoglobin in response to iron. The response to iron could not be related to the type of renal disease except that a rise in haemoglobin occurred in all patients with polycystic kidney disease; however, even in these patients the response was very variable. There was no correlation between the change in haemoglobin in response to iron therapy and either the duration of haemodialysis or the marrow iron stores. Thus patients with normal marrow iron stores were as likely to show a good response to iron as patients with low stores. No factor could be identified which was clearly associated with lack of improvement in anaemia although more severe blood loss could not be excluded as a cause since blood loss was not recorded accurately. Figure 9.4 shows the response to iron supplements in a female with polycystic kidney disease and illustrates the marked improvement in anaemia which is achieved in some patients. Prior to the onset of haemodialysis the haemoglobin was 11 g/dl and fell progressively to 6 g/dl after 28 weeks of haemodialysis, there being no major blood loss in this period. After treat-

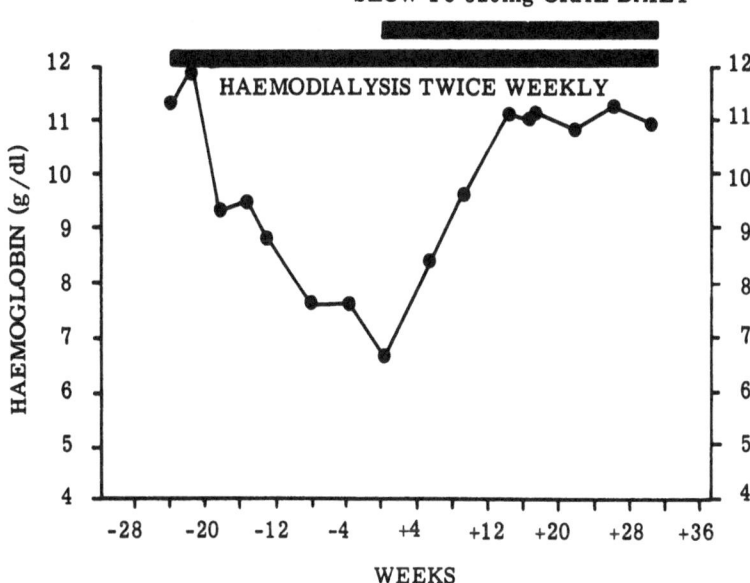

Figure 9.4   Response of anaemia to oral iron therapy in a female patient with polycystic kidney disease on haemodialysis

ment with oral iron, and without any alteration in dialysis regime, the haemoglobin rose progressively to 11 g/dl over the next 20 weeks.

These results confirm previous observations that a significant rise in haemoglobin in haemodialysis patients occurs following both oral[23, 28, 29] and intravenous iron supplements[25, 30-33] and as a result blood transfusion can be minimized – only three of the 28 patients in the study required blood transfusion during the 12-month period of iron therapy. In addition the results indicate that oral iron supplements are as effective as intravenous iron supplements, an important observation since in the past there has been controversy regarding the efficiency of iron absorption in chronic renal failure[24, 34, 35]. However, more recent studies indicate that iron absorption in chronic renal failure is normal and is regulated by the state of iron balance[36].

It is likely that the improvement in anaemia in response to iron is mainly due to correction of iron deficiency. However, in contrast to some previous observations[23, 25] there was a marked variation in the response irrespective of the initial iron status. The failure to predict the response of anaemia to iron therapy from the initial iron status may reflect both the limitations of the methods used to assess iron status and marked variation in blood loss. However, other factors may be involved in determining the response to iron in addition to iron status. In view of the known chronic blood loss in haemodialysis patients and, since the response to iron may be difficult to predict from the iron status, iron supplements should be given routinely to all haemodialysis patients.

When advocating long-term therapy the risk of iron overload must be considered. Marrow iron stores were reassessed in seven of our patients given oral iron and in nine given intravenous iron; after 12 months of treatment none developed high iron stores. Increased iron stores as indicated by serum ferritin have, however, been found after treatment with

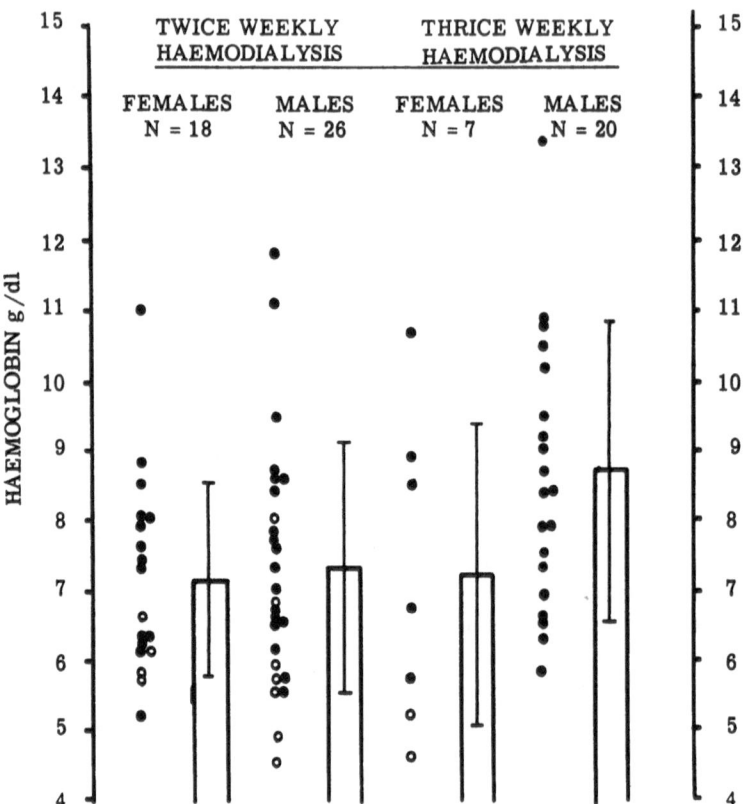

Figure 9.5   Effect of sex and frequency of haemodialysis on anaemia in haemodialysis patients. Closed circles indicate haemoglobin values for non transfused patients and open circles indicate values for patients who required blood transfusion in the previous year. The mean haemoglobin (± 1 SD) for each group is indicated by the column

intravenous iron for a longer period[27]. As the theoretical risk of inducing iron overload may be greater with intravenous than with oral iron the use of oral iron supplements may be safer on a long-term basis.

9.5 OTHER FACTORS INFLUENCING THE DEGREE OF ANAEMIA IN HAEMODIALYSIS PATIENTS

Sex, frequency of dialysis, the nature of the underlying renal disease and bilateral nephrectomy have all been reported to influence the degree of anaemia in haemodialysis patients.

9.5.1 Sex and frequency of dialysis

Figure 9.5 shows the haemoglobin in patients treated by haemodialysis twice and three times weekly according to sex. With haemodialysis for 6–8 h twice weekly there is no difference in haemoglobin in males compared to females and the proportion of patients requiring blood transfusion in each group is similar. In contrast in male patients treated by haemodialysis for 6 h three times weekly the haemoglobin is significantly higher than that both in males ($p < 0.02$) and females ($p < 0.02$) treated by haemodialysis twice weekly, and no patient required blood transfusion. In the limited number of females treated by haemodialysis for 6 h three times weekly the haemoglobin is in general no better than in those treated twice weekly. It has previously been suggested that anaemia is more severe in females than in males[1]. These results suggest that sex is not an important factor influencing anaemia on twice weekly haemodialysis. Improvement in anaemia with increased frequency of haemodialysis is well recognized[1]. However, our results suggest that increasing the frequency of haemodialysis produces a greater improvement in anaemia in males than females. That increasing the frequency of dialysis is of value in improving anaemia is confirmed when one looks at the change in haemoglobin in individual patients moving from twice to three times weekly haemodialysis (Figure 9.6). For the group as a whole there was a significant rise in haemoglobin with increasing frequency of dialysis. In individual patients the response was variable but a significant number of patients showed a beneficial rise in haemoglobin and this occurred in some females as well as males.

9.5.2 Nature of renal disease

Figure 9.7 shows the haemoglobin in our haemodialysis patients according to type of renal disease. Anaemia was least severe in patients with poly-

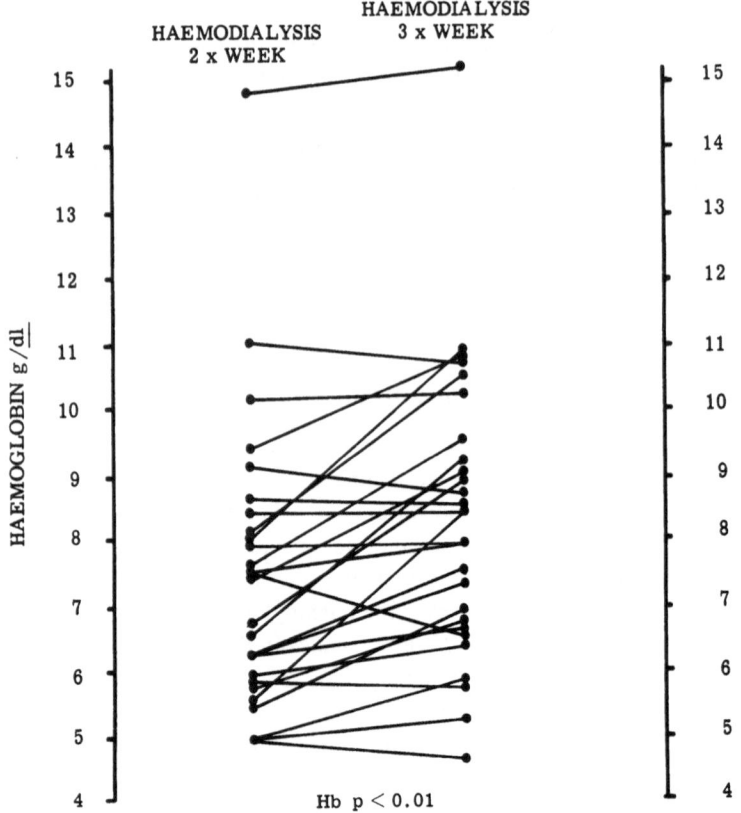

Figure 9.6   Change in haemoglobin in haemodialysis patients with increased frequency of haemodialysis. Haemoglobin values in individual patients on twice and thrice weekly haemodialysis are indicated by the closed circles, the two values being joined by a line

cystic kidney disease, the haemoglobin in this group being significantly higher than in patients with glomerulonephritis, pyelonephritis or hypertensive renal disease ($p < 0.001$) and this confirms previous similar findings[37]. Surprisingly, patients with congenital renal disease other than polycystic kidney disease had the next best haemoglobin although this was only significantly higher than that in patients with glomerulonephritis ($p < 0.05$). It has previously been suggested that patients with pyelonephritis and hypertensive renal disease are more severely anaemic than other patients[1]. However, we found no difference in the degree of anaemia in pyelonephritis compared to glomerulonephritis. Although the haemoglobin in patients with hypertensive renal disease was not significantly different to that in glomerulonephritis or pyelonephritis these patients

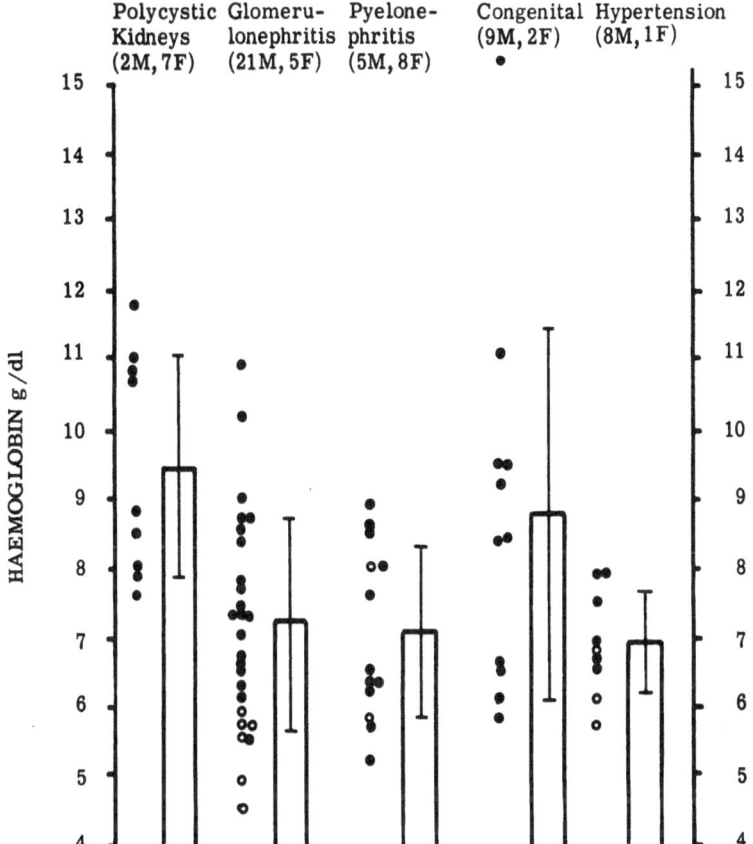

Figure 9.7   Haemoglobin in haemodialysis patients according to type of renal disease. Closed circles indicate haemoglobin values for non transfused patients and open circles indicate values for patients who required blood transfusion in the previous year. The mean haemoglobin ($\pm$ 1 SD) for each group is indicated by the column

seemed less capable of achieving more normal haemoglobin values. Thus the nature of the underlying renal disease may have some influence on the degree of anaemia and this could be related to residual erythropoietin secretion. In each disease type the range of haemoglobin values is wide so that residual erythropoietin secretion must vary widely within any disease type or there must be other factors involved.

9.5.3   Effect of bilateral nephrectomy

The deleterious effect of bilateral nephrectomy on anaemia in haemodialysis patients is well recognized, nephrectomized patients requiring twice the rate of blood transfusion as patients with intact renal tissue[8]. Figure 9.8 illustrates the catastrophic effect of bilateral nephrectomy on

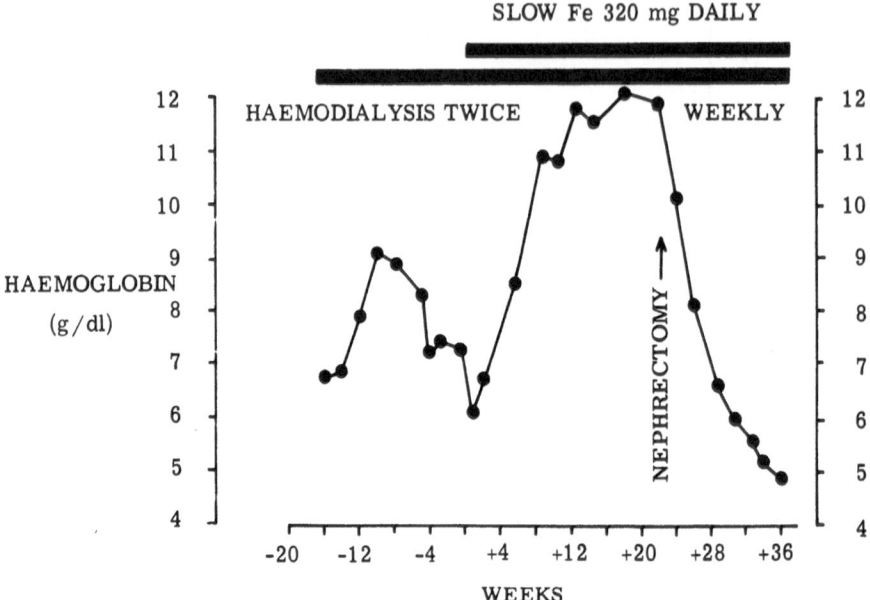

Figure 9.8   Effect of bilateral nephrectomy on anaemia in a male patient with polycystic kidney disease on haemodialysis

anaemia in a patient with polycystic kidney disease. Although this patient was anaemic following the commencement of regular haemodialysis the haemoglobin rose progressively towards normal after treatment with oral iron supplements. At this point bilateral nephrectomy was performed in preparation for renal transplantation and the haemoglobin thereafter fell progressively to 5 g/dl over 10 weeks and for the first time blood transfusion was required for symptomatic anaemia. The response in this patient stresses the role which damaged renal tissue plays in determining the degree of anaemia. Because of the resultant morbidity bilateral nephrectomy should never be performed in haemodialysis patients without very clear indications.

9.6 EFFECT OF ANDROGENS ON ANAEMIA IN HAEMODIALYSIS PATIENTS

The use of androgens in the treatment of renal anaemia has a good theoretical basis as is shown in Table 9.4[3]. A number of studies have demonstrated a significant improvement in anaemia in haemodialysis patients in response to parenteral androgens[38-41] the oral preparations having a less

TABLE 9.4   Effects of androgens on erythropoiesis

1. Stimulates endogenous production of erythropoietin by the kidney and possibly by extrarenal sources
2. Increases responsiveness of bone marrow to erythropoietin
3. Stimulates erythropoiesis *in vitro*

consistent effect[42, 43]. In some studies the irregular administration of parenteral iron may have influenced the results[38, 39] and one controlled study failed to show a significant benefit from androgen therapy[44]. More recently Von Hartitzsch and Kerr[32] have shown that the improvement in anaemia in response to androgens is no greater than that achieved with parenteral iron therapy. They also found that use of both together produced no greater effect than either used alone. There must, therefore, be doubt about the place of androgens in the treatment of anaemia in haemodialysis patients particularly since they may give rise to a number of adverse effects (Table 9.5) some of which are disturbing, especially to female patients. Figure 9.5 shows that the majority of haemodialysis patients given iron supplements can be maintained asymptomatic without severe anaemia and without the need for blood transfusion; it therefore seems unreasonable to subject these patients to the risk of troublesome effects of androgens. It has been suggested that androgens should be restricted to the small proportion of patients who, despite adequate dialysis and iron supplements, have persisting severe anaemia necessitating blood transfusion[1]. Included in this category are patients with refractory anaemia following bilateral nephrectomy. A significant improvement in anaemia

TABLE 9.5   Adverse effects of androgens

Virilization in females
Acne
Hyperlipidaemia
Priapism in males
Cholestatic jaundice

with reduction in blood transfusion requirements has been reported following treatment of anephric haemodialysis patients with androgens[38]. However, in general the response is less marked than in patients with intact kidneys and the results of treatment in some studies have been disappointing[32, 44].

9.7 COBALT CHLORIDE AS A TREATMENT OF REFRACTORY ANAEMIA FOLLOWING BILATERAL NEPHRECTOMY

Experimentally cobalt chloride stimulates erythropoietin secretion[13] and therefore might be of value in the treatment of anaemia in haemodialysis patients. In haemodialysis patients with refractory anaemia following bilateral nephrectomy a significant improvement in anaemia with reduction in blood transfusion requirements has been reported following treatment with cobalt chloride[45]. However, a number of side effects, some potentially serious, may occur during therapy[45] and the role of cobalt in the treatment of refractory anaemia is not clear.

9.8 BLOOD TRANSFUSION REQUIREMENTS IN HAEMODIALYSIS PATIENTS

Since 1970 we have restricted blood transfusion to a minimum, blood transfusion being given only for severe symptomatic anaemia or to replace major acute blood loss. Since 1972 all haemodialysis patients in Edinburgh have taken regular oral iron supplements. Table 9.6 shows the blood transfusion rate in our dialysis unit over the past 2 years. In both periods, approximately one third of patients treated by haemodialysis required

TABLE 9.6   Blood transfusion requirements in haemodialysis patients in Edinburgh

---

1.   *August 1975 to August 1976*
     – 50 patients treated for 329 patient months
     – 16 patients (32%) required blood transfusion
     – total blood transfused 55 units
     Transfusion rate 0.12 units/ patient month

2.   *August 1976 to April 1977*
     – 60 patients treated for 401 patient months
     – 21 patients (35%) required blood transfusion
     – total blood transfused 78 units
     Transfusion rate 0.17 units/ patient month

TABLE 9.7 Indications for blood transfusion in haemodialysis patients in Edinburgh. August 1976 to April 1977

1. Symptomatic Anaemia: 43 units given to 11 patients
   – 8 patients given 2 units or less
   – 3 patients given more than 2 units

2. *Replacement of blood loss during dialysis:* 2 units in 1 patient

3. *Medical and surgical complications:* 33 units given to 8 patients
   – post transplant rejection 4 units
   – pericardial effusion 8 units
   – bilateral nephrectomy (2 patients) 13 units
   – transplant nephrectomy 2 units
   – splenectomy 2 units
   – bleeding peptic ulcer 4 units

blood transfusion and the overall transfusion rate was only 0.1 unit per patient month.

Table 9.7 shows the indications for blood transfusion during the last year. Only 50% of the blood used in this period was given as treatment of symptomatic anaemia, and of the 11 patients in this category eight required 2 units or less while the remainder of the blood was required by the other three patients. Thus very few patients require regular blood transfusion for symptomatic anaemia. Only one patient required blood transfusion to replace acute blood loss during haemodialysis and this stresses the marked reduction in acute blood loss during haemodialysis in recent years. The remainder of the blood given in this period was required because of medical and surgical complications and this could not have been prevented.

As is illustrated in Figure 9.5, in the majority of haemodialysis patients, who are given a high protein intake with oral supplements of water soluble vitamins and iron, the haemoglobin can be maintained at a reasonable level without the need for blood transfusion, in a few patients the haemoglobin can be maintained at a nearly normal level while only in a small proportion is regular blood transfusion necessary.

References

1. Koch, K. M., Patyna, W. D., Shaldon, S. and Werner, E. (1974). Anaemia of the regular haemodialysis patient and its treatment. *Nephron*, 12, 405
2. Fried, W. (1975). Erythropoietin and the kidney. *Nephron*, 15, 327
3. Naets, J. P. (1975). Haematological disorders in renal failure. *Nephron*, 14, 181
4. Shaw, A. B. (1967). Haemolysis in chronic renal failure. *Br. Med. J.*, 2, 213

5. Desforges, J. F. and Dawson, J. P. (1958). The anemia of renal failure. *Arch. Intern. Med.*, 101, 326

6. Eschbach, J. W., Adamson, J. W. and Cook, J. D. (1970). Disorders of red blood cell production in uremia. *Arch. Intern. Med.*, 126, 812

7. Naets, J. P. and Heuse, A. F. (1962). Measurement of erythropoietin stimulating factor in anemic patients with and without renal lesions. *J. Lab. Clin. Med.*, 60, 365

8. Van Ypersele de Strihou, C. and Stragier, A. (1969). Effect of bilateral nephrectomy on transfusion requirements of patients undergoing chronic dialysis. *Lancet*, ii, 705

9. Fisher, J. W., Hatch, F. E., Roh, B. L., Allan, R. C. and Kelley, B. J. (1968). Erythropoietin inhibitor in kidney and plasma from anemic uremic human subjects. *Blood*, 31, 440

10. Markson, J. L. and Rennie, J. B. (1956). The anaemia of chronic renal insufficiency. The effect of serum from azotaemic patients on the maturation of normoblasts in suspension cultures. *Scot. Med. J.*, 1, 320

11. Eschbach, J. W. Jr., Funk, D., Adamson, J., Kuhn, I., Scribner, B. H. and Finch, C. A. (1967). Erythropoiesis in patients with renal failure undergoing chronic dialysis. *N. Engl. J. Med.*, 276, 653

12. Fried, W., Marver, D., Large, R. D. and Gurney, C. W. (1966). Studies on the erythropoietin stimulating factor in the plasma of mice after receiving testosterone. *J. Lab. Clin. Med.*, 68, 947

13. Goldwasser, E., Jacobson, L. O., Fried, W. and Plzak, L. (1958). Studies on erythropoiesis: V The effect of cobalt on the production of erythropoietin. *Blood*, 13, 55

14. Mann, D. L., Donati, R. M. and Gallagher, N. I. (1964). Erythropoietin assay and ferrokinetic measurements in anemic uremic patients. *J. Am. Med. Assoc.*, 194, 1321

15. Giordano, C., De Santo, N. G., Rinaldi, S., Acone, D., Eposito, R. and Gallo, B. (1973). Histidine for the treatment of uraemic anaemia. *Br. Med. J.*, 4, 716

16. Hartitzsch, B. Von, Carr, D., Kjellstrand, C. M. and Kerr, D. N. S. (1973). Normal red cell survival in well dialysed patients. *Trans. Am. Soc. Artif. Intern. Organs*, 19, 471

17. Botella, J., Traver, J. A., Sanz-Guajardo, D., Torres, M. T., Sanjuan, I. and Zabala, P. (1977). Chloramines, an aggravating factor in the anaemia of patients on regular dialysis treatment. *Proc. E.D.T.A.*, 14, 192 (London: Pitman

18. Hampers, C. L., Streiff, R., Nathan, D. G., Snyder, D. and Merrill, J. P. (1967). Megaloblastic hematopoiesis in uremia and in patients on long-term hemodialysis. *N. Engl. J. Med.*, 276, 551

19. Lindsay, R. M. and Burton, J. A. (1972). Blood loss from cannulation sites during haemodialysis. *Scot. Med. J.*, 17, 266

20. Hocken, A. G. and Marwah, P. K. (1971). Iatrogenic contribution to anaemia of chronic renal failure. *Lancet*, i, 164

21. Lindsay, R. M. and Kennedy, A. C. (1972). Dialysers and blood loss in regular dialysis therapy. *Proc. E.D.T.A.*, 9, 437 (London: Pitman Medical)

22. Curtis, J. R., Eastwood, J. B., Smith, E. K. M., Storey, J. M., Verroust, P. J., De Wardener, H. E., Wing, A. J. and Wolfson, E. M. (1969). Maintenance haemodialysis. *Q. J. Med.*, 61, 49

23. Baker, L. R. I., Cattell, W. R., Child, J. A. and Saudie, E. (1975). Iron therapy in maintenance haemodialysis. *Clin. Sci.*, **48**, 529

24. Eschbach, J. W., Cook, J. D. and Finch, C. A. (1970). Iron absorption in chronic renal disease. *Clin. Sci.*, **38**, 191

25. Morgan, T. (1972). The effect of intravenous iron on the haematocrit of patients on maintenance haemodialysis. *Med. J. Aust.*, **1**, 852

26. Beutler, E., Robson, M. J. and Buttenwieser, E. (1958). A comparison of the plasma iron, iron-binding capacity, sternal marrow iron and other methods in the clinical evaluation of iron stores. *Ann. Intern. Med.*, **48**, 60

27. Hussein, S., Priesto, J., O'Shea, M., Hoffbrand, A. V., Baillod, R. A. and Moorhead, J. F. (1975). Serum ferritin assay and iron status in chronic renal failure and haemodialysis. *Br. Med. J.*, **1**, 546

28. Wallace, M. R. (1971). The effect of oral iron on the anaemia of patients on maintenance haemodialysis. *N.Z. Med. J.*, **74**, 167

29. Strickland, I. D., Chaput de Saintonge, D. M., Boulton, F. E., Brain, A. J. S., Goodwin, F. J., Marsh, F. P. and Zychova, Z. (1974). A trial of oral iron in dialysis patients. *Clin. Nephrol.*, **21**, 13

30. Carter, R. A., Hawkins, J. B. and Robinson, B. H. B. (1969). Iron metabolism in the anaemia of chronic renal failure. Effects of dialysis and of parenteral iron. *Br. Med. J.*, **3**, 206

31. Stewart, W. K., Fleming, L. W. and Shepherd, A. M. M. (1976). Haemoglobin and serum iron responses to periodic intravenous iron-dextran infusions during maintenance dialysis. *Nephron*, **17**, 121

32. Hartitzsch, B. Von and Kerr, D. N. S. (1976). Response to parenteral iron with and without androgen therapy in patients undergoing regular haemodialysis. *Nephron*, **17**, 430

33. Wright, F. K., Goldsmith, H. J. and Hall, S. M. (1968). Iron responsive anaemia in repeated dialysis treatment without routine blood transfusion. *Proc. E.D.T.A.*, **5**, 179 (Amsterdam: Excerpta Medica Foundation)

34. Brozovich, B., Cattell, W. R., Cottrall, M. F., Gwyther, M. M., McMillan, J. M., Malpas, J. S., Salsbury, A. and Trott, N. G. (1971). Iron metabolism in patients undergoing regular dialysis therapy. *Br. Med. J.*, **1**, 695

35. Lawson, D. H., Boddy, K., King, P. C., Lenton, A. L. and Will, G. (1971). Iron metabolism in patients with chronic renal failure on regular dialysis treatment. *Clin. Sci.*, **41**, 345

36. Milman, N. and Larsen, L. (1976). Iron absorption in patients with chronic uraemia undergoing regular haemodialysis. *Acta Med. Scand.*, **199**, 113

37. Maggiore, Q., Navelesi, R., Biagini, M., Balestre, P. L. and Giagnoni, P. (1967). Comparative studies of uraemic anaemia in polycystic kidney disease and in other renal diseases. *Proc. E.D.T.A.*, **4**, 264 (Amsterdam: Excerpta Medica Foundation)

38. Shaldon, S., Koch, K. M., Oppermann, F., Patyna, W. D. and Schoeppe, W. (1971). Testosterone therapy for anaemia in maintenance haemodialysis. *Br. Med. J.*, **3**, 212

39. Hendler, E. D., Goffinet, J. A., Ross, S., Longnecker, R. E. and Bakovic, V. (1974). Controlled study of androgen therapy in anemia of patients on maintenance hemodialysis. *N. Engl. J. Med.*, **291**, 1046

40. Williams, J. S., Stein, J. H. and Ferris, T. M. (1974). Nandrolone Deconate therapy for patients receiving hemodialysis. *Arch. Intern. Med.*, **134**, 289

41. Hartitzbch, B. Von, Kerr, D. N. S., Morley, G. and Marks, B. (1977). Androgens in the anaemia of chronic renal failure. *Nephron*, **18**, 13
42. Davies, M., Muckle, T. J., Cassells-Smith, A., Webster, D. and Kerr, D. N. S. (1972). Oxymethalone in the treatment of anaemia in chronic renal failure. *Br. J. Urol.*, **44**, 387
43. Lindholm, D. D., Fisher, J. W., Vieira, J. A., Dombeck, D. H., Bernal, G. and Lerthora, J. (1973). Clinical effects of oral fluoxymesterone in patients with dialysis-controlled uremia. *Trans. Am. Soc. Artif. Intern. Organs*, **19**, 475
44. Ball, J. H., Lowrie, E. G., Hampers, C. L. and Merrill, J. P. (1975). Testosterone therapy in hemodialysis patients. *Clin. Nephrol.*, **4**, 91
45. Duckham, J. M. and Lee, H. A. (1976). The treatment of refractory anaemia of chronic renal failure with cobalt chloride. *Q. J. Med.*, **69**, 277

DISCUSSION

A. W. Siemsen (Honolulu): Were Winney's patients taken off antacids?

Winney: No, they were not.

Siemsen: There is considerable evidence that antacids do bind oral iron. There have been several studies that showed that it does not respond quite so well, and one reason was that the patients were on oral antacid.

Winney: Our patients also took ascorbic acid, and that may have had some effect on the absorption of iron. They do take them, and we did get a response, but whether there is a variation in response is something that could be looked at further.

They were taking their antacids.

J. S. Cameron: And what about oral vitamins, including pyrodixine?

Winney: Yes.

C. P. Swainson (Edinburgh): There is a relationship with the time of day when they are taken. Vitamins and similar substances are usually taken fasting, before breakfast, whereas aluminium binders and phosphate binders are usually taken before meals. There might be an effect from that.

R. Gabriel (London): How were haemoglobin measurements standardized, and were red cell masses done in these people.

Winney: I cannot answer the point on standardization of haemoglobin without asking the haematologist. Red cell masses were not done.

B. H. B. Robinson (Birmingham): We did some work a few years back on red cell masses and we measured the haemoglobin in dialysis patients and we were surprised to find how well they correlated in that the haemoglobin really did seem to relate to changes in red cell mass.

157

Since it now looks as though it will be mandatory upon us to transfuse the patients who are to have transplants, how will this affect our approach to the management of renal anaemia?

Winney: From the point of view of the patients, in terms of their own management, particularly those with polycystic kidneys, it would be unethical to give them blood transfusions and prevent them from achieving a normal haemoglobin level from their own marrow. Regular transfusions have been shown to be one of the factors depressing readings in these patients. I find that very difficult.

Robinson: But there are a number of people who would consider it unethical to transplant somebody who had not had a transfusion.

J. S. Robson (Edinburgh): The number of transfusions required to achieve the immunological advantage is very small so it might not affect the overall haematological position very much.

10

Mineral metabolism in chronic renal failure
J. A. Kanis

10.1   INTRODUCTION

Since the advent of dialysis and renal transplantation, patients with end-stage chronic renal disease are surviving for long periods of time, whereas formerly they would have died. Of the many disorders that affect such survivors, much attention has been directed to disturbances in mineral metabolism. Advances in the past few years, particularly in the field of vitamin D metabolism, have led to an understanding of some of the pathogenic processes which give rise to these disorders. The 'spin-off' has been that, despite the complexity of the disorders, the objectives of treatment and the ways in which these objectives might be realized, have become clearer.

This report considers mainly the problems which are encountered in advanced renal failure. For a wider appraisal of the subject the reader is referred to a number of reviews[1-4].

10.2   DEFINITION AND PREVALENCE OF RENAL BONE DISEASE

The skeletal disorders which are found in chronic renal failure (Table 10.1) may occur singly or in various combinations. None of these disorders is however unique to renal disease and none is specific to a particular population of patients such as those managed conservatively, those on haemodialysis or indeed transplanted patients. There are, however, differences in the prevalence of the various abnormalities not only within these population sub-groups but also between renal units[5-7]. Some of these differences reflect the use of differing criteria for the diagnosis of bone disease.

Bone disease is frequently a major clinical problem in the young[8], particularly at the time of skeletal maturity, when requirements for vitamin

TABLE 10.1   Features of renal bone disease. Metastatic calcification may be the result of disturbed mineral metabolism but cannot be considered a skeletal disorder except in the ectopic calcification of cartilage (e.g. pseudogout) and osteoid

Retardation of growth
Osteomalacia and rickets
Osteitis fibrosa
Osteosclerosis
Periosteal new bone formation
Osteoporosis
Osteonecrosis
Metastatic calcification

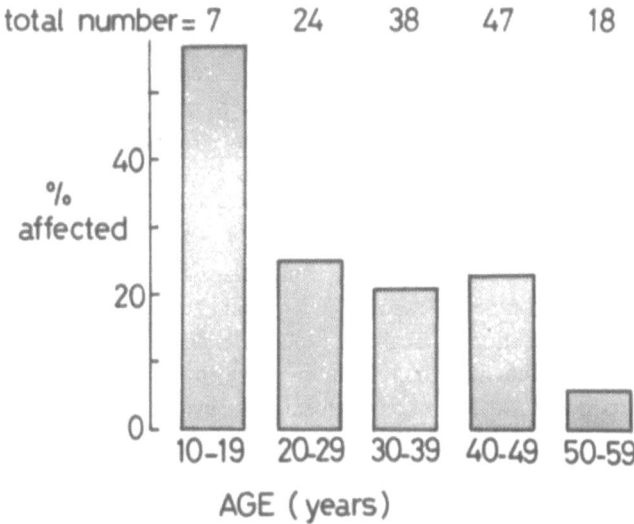

Figure 10.1   Prevalence of subperiosteal erosions on x-ray examination in 134 patients about to start treatment with haemodialysis

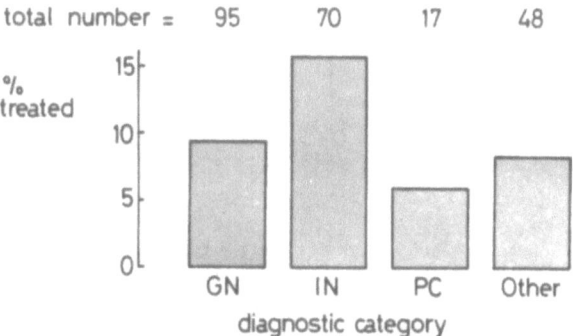

Figure 10.2   Prevalence of osteitis fibrosa associated with bone pain in 230 patients established on dialysis treatment. Patients were subdivided according to the nature of their renal disorder (GN, glomerulonephritis; IN, interstitial nephropathy, i.e. chronic pyelonephritis and analgesic nephropathy; PC, polycystic disease; the term 'other' includes patients in whom the diagnosis was doubtful). Affected patients were selected for treatment with D-metabolites. A greater proportion of patients with interstitial nephropathy required treatment than was necessary in patients with other renal diseases

D may be the greatest. The prevalence of osteitis fibrosa at end-stage renal disease is highest in this age group and decreases progressively with age (Figure 10.1). Patients with interstitial forms of renal disease may also be more susceptible[9,10] (Figure 10.2) which might reflect a comparatively longer duration of uraemia compared to patients with other forms of renal disease. An alternative explanation might be that damage to interstitial tissue destroys tubular sites responsible for the production of vitamin D metabolites or for the degradation of parathyroid hormone. Other factors which affect the incidence of renal bone disease include geographical variation and environmental factors[5-7, 11, 12], but the mechanisms by which these factors cause bone disease are obscure. Recent advances in our understanding of the disturbances in metabolism that occur in chronic renal failure have resulted in the proposal that several 'pathophysiological pathways' may be of prime importance.

10.3 PATHOGENESIS OF RENAL BONE DISEASE

Two of the concepts of the pathogenesis of renal bone disease have been popularized in recent years. The first holds that hyperparathyroidism and

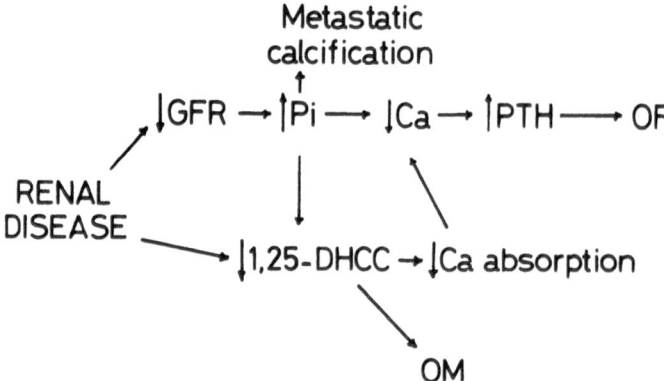

Figure 10.3. Schematic flow diagram to show current hypotheses for the pathogenesis of renal bone disease. Renal disease results in progressive decrements in glomerular filtration rate (GFR) and in the ability to synthesize 1,25-dihydroxycholecalciferol (1,25-DHCC). An increase in plasma phosphate (Pi), due to a fall in GFR, stimulates the secretion of parathyroid hormone (PTH) indirectly by decreasing plasma levels of calcium (Ca). Because of the biological effects of PTH, plasma levels of Ca and Pi tend toward normal at the expense of increased secretion of PTH and osteitis fibrosa (OF) until the decrease in GFR outstrips the compensatory capabilities of PTH. Hyperphosphataemia may further inhibit synthesis of 1,25-DHCC. Malabsorption of calcium may contribute to secondary hyperparathyroidism, and a deficiency of D induce osteomalacia (OM)

its skeletal consequences (osteitis fibrosa) is the result of phosphate retention. The other proposes that defective production of 1,25-dihydroxy-cholecalciferol by the kidney results in malabsorption of calcium and defective mineralization of bone (osteomalacia). These hypotheses are not mutually exclusive (Figure 10.3).

10.3.1 Phosphate metabolism

Elegant animal experiments[13,14] have demonstrated that incremental restriction of dietary phosphate, in proportion to decrements induced in glomerular filtration rate, may abolish the secondary stimulation of secretion of parathyroid hormone. The hypothesis derived from these experiments holds that a rise in plasma phosphate due to impaired renal function, results in a decrease in the ionized fraction of plasma calcium and thus stimulates the secretion of parathyroid hormone. The increase in circulating parathyroid hormone so induced, reduces the renal tubular reabsorption of phosphate, so that any increase in plasma levels of phosphate due to chronic renal failure is minimized. The maintenance of a near normal plasma level of phosphate, together with the calcaemic effects of parathyroid hormone (increased bone resorption and renal tubular reabsorption of calcium), mean that disturbances in the ionized fraction of plasma calcium are also minimal. Thus, during the course of progressive renal failure, plasma levels of calcium and phosphate remain relatively normal but at the expense of an ever-increasing secretion rate of parathyroid hormone. When the decrement in filtration is too great to be compensated by the renal effects of parathyroid hormone, hyperphosphataemia and hypocalcaemia accompany high levels of parathyroid hormone.

The importance of this pathogenic mechanism in man is perhaps supported by finding increased circulating levels of parathyroid hormone and an inverse relationship between plasma calcium and phosphate in patients in the early stages of chronic renal failure[15,16]. In addition, the administration of phosphate to healthy subjects may reduce plasma calcium levels and increase those of parathyroid hormone. There is however conflicting evidence as to the effects of chronic manipulation of plasma phosphate on the secretion of parathyroid hormone in man[16-18]. Moreover, in chronic renal failure, raised plasma levels of parathyroid hormone might be due to its impaired degradation by the kidney. Irrespective of the mechanisms by which levels of parathyroid hormone are increased, it is not certain whether the hormone is circulating in an active form, since measurements made using radioimmunoassay might not reflect biological activity.

Phosphate is also an important factor in the mineralization of bone.

There is a striking negative correlation between prevailing levels of plasma phosphate and the amount of non-mineralized osteoid in patients with chronic renal failure and in patients with normal renal function[5,19,20]. This relationship is not necessarily dependent on vitamin D status or on renal function since the correlation is observed in dialysis patients (Figure 10.4);

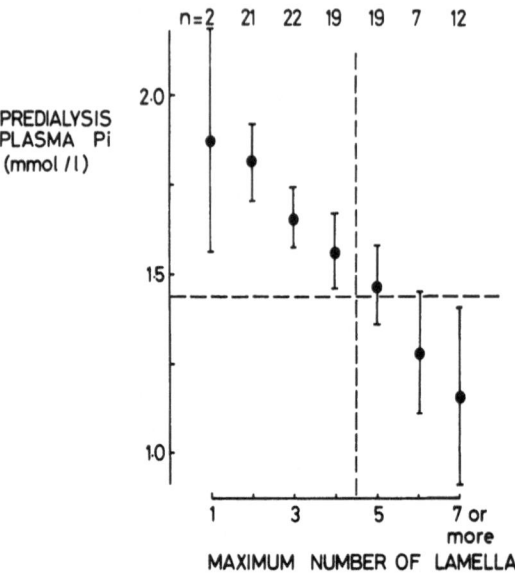

Figure 10.4 Relationship between plasma phosphate (mean of values taken immediately before a dialysis treatment ± SEM) and the number of osteoid lamellae seen in histological sections. Osteomalacia (five or more lamellae) was uncommon in patients with high levels of plasma phosphate. Evidence of osteomalacia was commonly noted in patients whose plasma phosphate lay below the upper limit for the normal range (horizontal dashed line). (From Kanis *et al.*[5])

and in Pagetic patients, it exists independently of circulating levels of 25-hydroxy-vitamin D_3. The causal significance of this relationship is suggested by observations in patients with or without renal disease that phosphate restriction may induce and phosphate repletion may cure defective mineralization of bone[11,21]. The levels of plasma phosphate in patients with chronic renal failure below which osteomalacia may be induced are considerably higher than those associated with defective mineralization in patients with normal renal function.

10.3.2 Vitamin D metabolism

Disturbed metabolism of vitamin D may be an important additional factor in the pathogenesis of osteomalacia and hyperparathyroidism in chronic renal failure. It is well recognized that large but unphysiological doses of vitamin D_2 or D_3 may increase the intestinal absorption of calcium and improve osteomalacia and osteitis fibrosa in such patients[22]. This resistance to vitamin D (in the sense that doses of vitamin required to effect a biological response are much greater than the physiological requirements necessary to maintain the integrity of the normal skeleton) is thought to be due to defective metabolism of vitamin D. The kidney may be the major site of synthesis of dihydroxylated metabolites of vitamin D (1,25-dihydroxycholecalciferol and 24,25-dihydroxycholecalciferol)[23-25]. The development of bone disease and D-resistance of patients with chronic renal disease may result in part from impaired endogenous production of these hormones[23-26]. Production of 1,25-dihydroxycholecalciferol is defective in patients with advanced chronic renal disease, and the absence of this hormonal form of vitamin D has been considered to contribute in large measure to the D-resistance and bone disease of such patients. However, long-term administration of $l\alpha$-hydroxylated metabolites of vitamin D does not always result in an improvement in bone disease, and apparently favourable biochemical responses may be associated with demineralization and occasionally with deterioration of pre-existing bone disease[10,27,28]. Patients with severe renal impairment, including anephric patients, do not necessarily have bone disease nor does this inevitably develop with time[5]. These observations suggest that factors, other than defective renal production of 1,25-dihydroxy vitamin D_3 may be at least as important. Preliminary studies showing effects of 24,25-dihydroxycholecalciferol on retention of calcium, mineralization, and cartilage metabolism suggest that deficiency of this hormone in chronic renal failure may also be important in the production of bone disease.

10.3.3 Other factors

Renal failure is associated with the retention of potential toxins such as indoles, guanidines, phenols, aliphatic amines and other 'middle molecules' which are yet to be identified[29,30]. Substances normally found in trace amounts such as fluoride[12], aluminium[31], vitamin A[32,33] and cadmium[34] may also accumulate and contribute to disordered mineral metabolism. Disturbances in acid-base balance[35-36] and in the metabolism of hormones other than parathyroid hormone and vitamin D occur in chronic renal failure. Affected hormones include calcitonin, growth hormone, sex hormones, prolactin and thyroid hormone, all of which may variously affect skeletal tissue itself or the metabolism of its regulating hormones[37-41]. The relative importance of these factors is controversial and, at present, their relevance in modifying approaches to treatment is uncertain.

10.4 PATHOGENESIS OF ECTOPIC CALCIFICATION

Though collagen promotes the precipitation of calcium and phosphate *in vitro*, the physiological mechanisms which initiate the formation and growth of mineral crystals and the factors which inhibit these processes in various connective tissues are unknown. In chronic renal failure the additional factors controlling soft-tissue calcification are also unclear,

TABLE 10.2   Clinical manifestations of disturbed mineral metabolism in chronic renal failure

	Disorders	*Clinical consequences*
1.	Hyperparathyroidism and osteitis fibrosa	Skeletal deformity Bone pain Pruritis
2.	Osteomalacia and decreased availability of vitamin D and phosphate	Skeletal deformity Bone pain Pathological fracture Proximal myopathy Haemolytic anaemia
3.	Osteoporosis	Pathological fracture Skeletal deformity
4.	Osteonecrosis	Joint pain Osteoarthrosis
5.	Osteosclerosis and periosteal new bone formation	None known
6.	Ectopic calcification (*a*) Periarticular (*b*) Skin and eye (*c*) Vascular (*d*) Visceral	 Joint pain and limitation of movement Pruritis, red eye syndrome, corneal calcification Limitation of vascular access sites (including those required for transplantation). Vascular insufficiency of skin and muscle. ? Atheroma Heart block, cardiac failure, respiratory failure

though disturbed metabolism of collagen, pyrophosphate and magnesium may be important. From clinical observation[4,42] it is clear that the availability of calcium and phosphate are of direct importance, which is hardly surprising since they are invariable constituents of ectopic deposits. Ectopic calcification may be induced by the use of dialysate solutions rich in calcium or by increasing the intestinal absorption of calcium with vitamin D[43,44]. Fluctuations in plasma phosphate are generally greater than those seen in calcium[4], and changes in the availability of phosphate must be quantitatively more important than those of calcium.

Symptoms of ectopic calcification depend upon the tissues which are involved (Table 10.2). Symptoms and the deposits themselves may improve following restriction of dietary phosphate, or measures which reduce the balance of calcium. The possible importance of parathyroid hormone is suggested by the improvements in pruritis, periarticular or vascular calcification which may follow parathyroidectomy[4], though it is difficult to dissociate effects attributable to removal of parathyroid hormone itself from consequential changes in mineral metabolism.

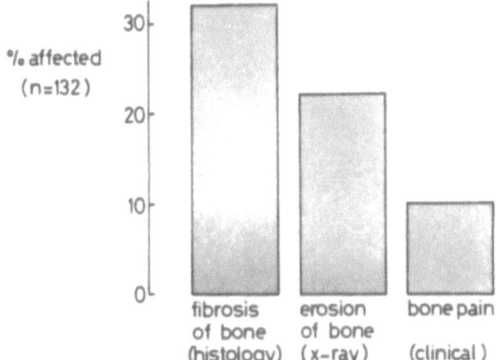

Figure 10.5 The prevalence of hyperparathyroidism in 132 patients with end-stage chronic renal failure about to start treatment with long-term haemodialysis. The prevalence depends upon the diagnostic criteria used and the methods of assessment. Histological abnormalities (marrow fibrosis) are more frequent than radiographic abnormalities. Symptoms occur in a minority.

10.5 FEATURES OF RENAL BONE DISEASE

Though renal bone disease is common, symptoms arising directly from skeletal disease itself are unusual[4] (Figure 10.5). But underlying biochemical disorders giving rise to bone disease may also express themselves clinically (Table 10.2).

10.5.1   Osteitis fibrosa

Histological features include the deposition of excessive amounts of fibrous tissue in the marrow spaces. This is associated with an increase in the numbers of active looking bone cells (osteoclasts and osteoblasts). Plasma levels of parathyroid hormone, alkaline phosphatase, and hydroxyproline are higher than those found in patients without fibrosis and provide useful biochemical markers of disease activity[45]. Subperiosteal resorption of bone is the characteristic radiographic feature, but is less commonly seen than abnormalities in histology of bone (Figure 10.5). In some instances, particularly in children, erosions may give rise to skeletal deformities (Figure 10.6). Bone pain is uncommon (Figure 10.5).

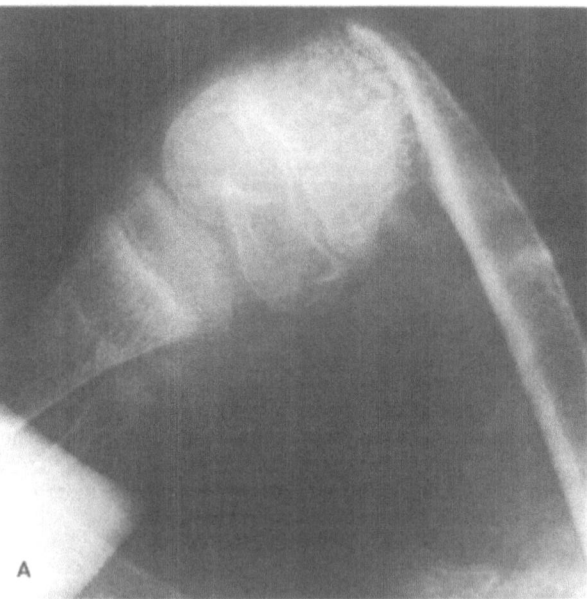

Figure 10.6   Radiographic features of renal bone disease. (A) Subperiosteal bone resorption in a child with renal failure. Resorption has caused deformity of the femur (from Kanis *et al.*[45])

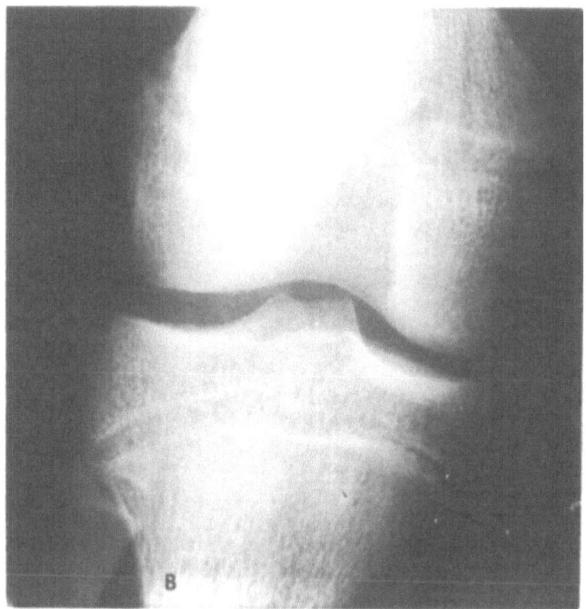

Figure 10.6 (B) Appearances similar to rickets in the tibia of a child with untreated renal bone disease (from Kanis *et al.*[45])

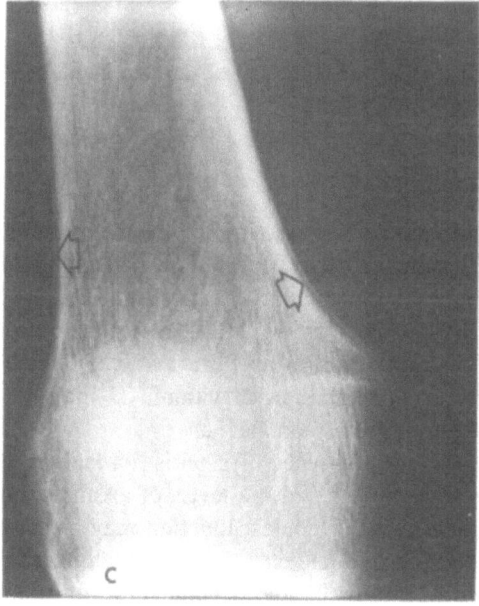

Figure 10.6 (C) Periosteal new bone formation. The periosteal separation from the mineralized cortex of the femur is shown by the arrows

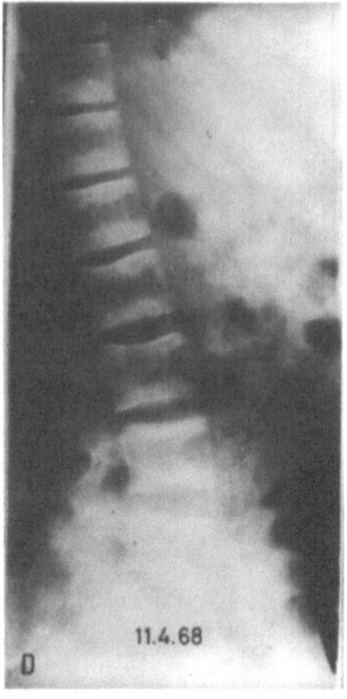

Figure 10.6   (D) Osteosclerosis of the spine. Alternate bands of sclerosis give rise to a 'rugger jersey' appearance

10.5.2   Osteomalacia

In chronic renal disease an increase in the amount of unmineralized bone (osteoid) may reflect its increased formation, defective mineralization or both. The incidence of osteomalacia varies enormously between renal units. In Oxford its incidence is low and does not increase with the duration of dialysis treatment even in anephric patients[5] which suggests that defective production of metabolites of vitamin D may not be the major factor in the pathogenesis of osteomalacia.

Bone cell counts, in the absence of osteitis fibrosa, are commonly low and, unlike nutritional rickets, plasma levels of alkaline phosphatase may be normal[46]. In some cases osteoblast function may be suppressed by low levels of plasma phosphate induced by over-zealous administration of phosphate binding agents or by the accumulation of aluminium. Radiographic abnormalities, similar to those found in D-deficient disorders (Figure 10.6) are relatively uncommon and bone biopsy, rather than x-rays or plasma measurements, may be the most powerful diagnostic aid. *In vivo* neutron activation analysis to measure total body or spinal calcium may provide a sensitive indirect index of response to treatment[27], but this technique is not widely available.

10.5.3 Osteosclerosis and periosteal new bone formation

These disorders are due to an increase in bone matrix either below the periosteal surface or in trabecular bone. These disorders are usually diagnosed by their characteristic x-ray appearances (Figure 10.6)[47] since they do not give rise to clinical problems. Osteosclerosis and periosteal new bone formation may be induced in experimental animals by the infusion of high doses of parathyroid hormone[48] but in patients with chronic renal failure they may be associated more with osteomalacia, where levels of parathyroid hormone are characteristically lower[49] than with osteitis fibrosa. Osteosclerosis may be seen for the first time on x-ray when osteomalacia is effectively treated with vitamin D.

10.5.4 Osteoporosis

A reduction in bone mass is commonly observed in chronic renal disease but is associated with abnormalities in bone matrix[1]. For this reason the term osteopaenia is sometimes used to distinguish the disorder from osteoporosis which by definition presupposes normality of collagen matrix. Osteoporosis is commonly progressive in patients on dialysis treatment[50] and the rate of bone loss may be accelerated for a short time after transplantation[51]. Its aetiology is unknown but factors of possible importance include the level of calcium used in the dialysis fluid, the administration of drugs which include steroids, cytotoxic agents and heparin as well as alterations in the metabolism of vitamin D[51,52].

10.5.5 Avascular necrosis

Avascular necrosis occurs most commonly when steroids are used in the treatment of the underlying renal disorder (especially transplantation). It is likely that the combination of steroids and chronic renal failure are additive risk factors, since its occurrence is uncommon in steroid-treated patients without chronic renal failure or rarely noted in patients with renal impairment who are untreated with steroids. The pathogenesis of avascular necrosis is unknown and this is reflected by the increasing number of causative factors which have been invoked[53]. The disorder may be symptomless but pain is frequently present, which is presumably due to progressive necrosis, collapse of bone and secondary osteoarthrosis.

10.5.6 Metastatic calcification

The prevalence and effects of metastatic calcification are aspects of mineral metabolism that have been less well studied than others. This is due to the difficulties with which it is diagnosed in its early stages and its uncertain contribution to mortality and morbidity. In patients with florid ectopic calcification, it may give rise to serious disability and death (Table 10.2), but more frequently it presents as an incidental finding on radiographs and cannot be directly implicated in the morbidity of affected patients. It is however possible that calcification in blood vessels, even to an extent which is undetectable by x-ray techniques, may have important clinical consequences. For example, in patients with chronic renal failure, the risk of death and morbidity from atherosclerotic vascular disease may be greater than that of the healthy population[54]. Whilst risk factors such as hyperlipidaemia and hypertension may be important in this respect, the role of disturbed mineral metabolism might also be important in the regulation of platelet function or in the growth of atherosclerotic plaques. Observations that the diphosphonates, inhibitors, of mineralization and crystal growth, may prevent the induction of atheroma in animals fed atherogenic diets, give some credence to this view.

The factors which operate to give rise to calcification at various non-skeletal sites may well differ since periarticular lesions are commonly improved by restriction of dietary phosphate or by parathyroidectomy[4], but their effects on vascular, ectodermal and visceral calcification are less predictable (Figure 10.7).

10.6 TREATMENT

Treatment strategy should be based not only on the nature of the skeletal disorder but also on a careful assessment of the biochemical abnormalities by which the disorder arose. The likely management of the chronic renal disease itself should also be considered since, for example, therapeutic approaches may depend on the probability of subsequent transplantation.

10.6.1 Prophylaxis

There are a number of preventative measures which should be considered in all patients with advanced renal impairment. It is probable that the

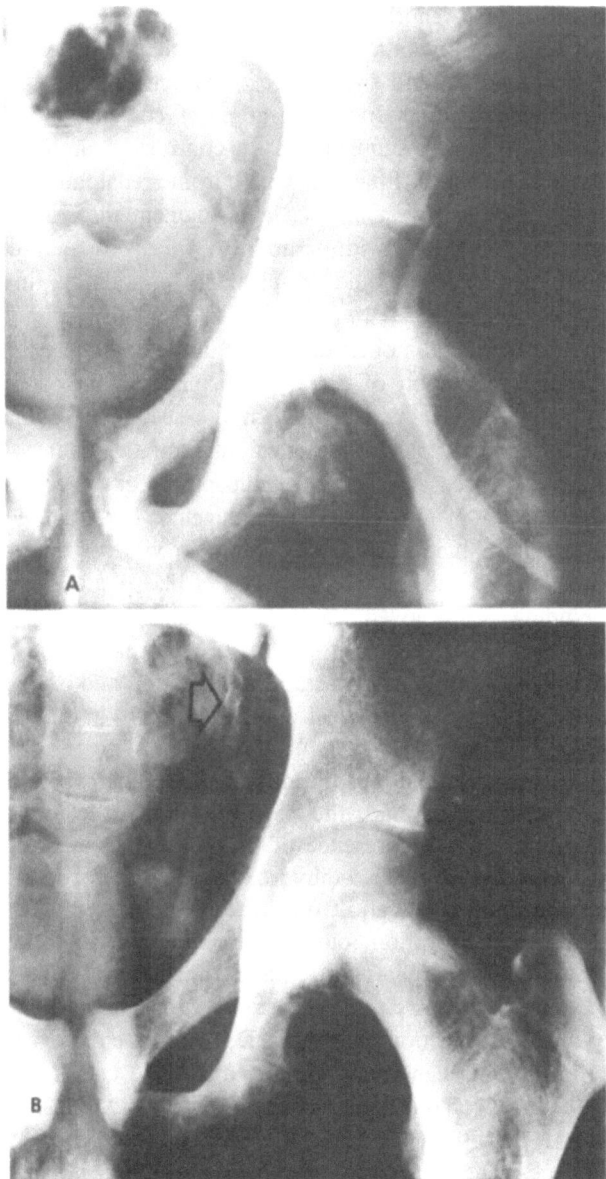

Figure 10.7 Metastatic (periatricular and vascular) calcification and erosions of bone in a patient treated by intermittent haemodialysis (A). X-rays taken 6 months after subtotal parathyroidectomy (B) show regression of erosions and soft tissue deposits but persistence of vascular calcification (arrow)

restriction of dietary intake of protein, as currently practised, is a greater factor in the induction of morbidity than it is in achieving beneficial effects. With respect to mineral metabolism, protein deficient diets tend to restrict the intake of vitamin C and pyridoxine[55,56] which both act as essential co-factors in the formation and maturation of collagen. These factors should be given as dietary supplements. In contrast, vitamin A accumulates, at least in the plasma of patients with chronic renal failure[55]. Vitamin A may cause bone resorption *in vitro* and augment the release of para-thyroid hormone. Overdose with vitamin A *in vivo* may induce bone disease and hypercalcaemia, and supplements containing this vitamin should therefore be avoided.

Unlike the experimental models developed in the dog, there is at present no evidence that restriction of dietary phosphate in proportion to the degree of renal insufficiency, will prevent the secondary stimulation of parathyroid hormone. It is not practical to limit the dietary intake of phosphate but decreased availability of phosphate for absorption can be achieved with the use of phosphate-binding agents. These should be given to avoid the risks of metastatic calcification. In view of the association between osteomalacia and low plasma levels of phosphate, the amount of phosphate-binding drugs given should be regulated according to their effects on plasma phosphate. The level of predialysis plasma phosphate that best balances the risks of metastatic calcification and osteomalacia is unknown but probably lies between 1.6 and 2.2 mmol/l in dialysis patients (Figure 10.4).

Unlike the net intestinal absorption of phosphate which is largely dependent on the dietary load, the net absorption of calcium is more critically dependent on the presence of the vitamin D metabolites. It is thought that deficiency of 1,25-dihydroxycholecalciferol, which results from damage to renal tissue and from hyperphosphataemia, is the cause for the calcium malabsorption found in uraemia. But in some patients, especially those not yet on dialysis treatment, deficiency of this metabolite may also be due to low plasma levels of 25-hydroxycholecalciferol[57] induced by dietary restriction of vitamin D, imposed either by the patient or the physician. This can easily be remedied. The use of drugs which interfere with the metabolism or action of vitamin D, such as steroids, phenytoin and barbiturates[58] should, where possible, be avoided. In patients with end-stage renal disease, in whom the dietary intake of vitamin D is adequate, defective renal production of 1,25-dihydroxycholecalciferol probably accounts, in large measure, for the malabsorption of calcium. In such cases net absorption of calcium can be augmented by increases in the dietary intake but massive doses are required[59]. Unless the diet is deficient in calcium, increases in absorption are more readily induced with the use of vitamin D. Vitamin D and its metabolites will increase intestinal absorption of calcium and increase the plasma concentration. At present, the prophylactic use of these agents in preventing defective mineralization or secondary hyperparathyroidism is not established, though they may be effective in the prevention of osteopaenia or in the treatment of established bone disease.

The dialysis membrane provides a site for the loss or the incorporation of calcium into the body. The net transfer is dependent on shifts in plasma pH and protein levels, and on the respective calcium concentrations of plasma and dialysis fluid. The use of a low dialysate calcium (1.25 mmol/l) may aggravate osteopaenia but might also decrease the risk of metastatic calcification[52]. The use of calcium rich dialysis fluids (2.00 mmol/l) is not advised, despite reports of decreased secretion of parathyroid hormone[60], since metastatic calcification may be accentuated and the skeletal response disappointing[43]. As in the case of optimum levels of plasma phosphate, the ideal calcium concentration of dialysis fluid is unknown. Observations using a variety of techniques suggest that osteopaenia does not follow the use of dialysis fluids with a calcium level of 1.63 to 1.75 mmol/l[52,61].

10.6.2 Established bone disease

The administration of vitamin D, 25-hydroxy-, 1α-hydroxy- and 1,25-dihydroxy vitamin D may all increase plasma calcium, augment the balance and intestinal absorption of calcium and phosphate, and suppress the secretion of parathyroid hormone[10,22,45] (Figure 10.8). The rationale for their use in bone disease is based on the supposition that a decrease in the secretion of parathyroid hormone will reverse osteitis fibrosa and that the effects of the vitamin itself on target tissues will directly or indirectly induce normal mineralization. In practice, symptoms regress in the majority of patients but histological improvements are less consistently seen[10,28]. It is not yet known whether patients who fail to respond to vitamin D$_2$ or D$_3$ will respond more favourably to 1α-hydroxylated metabolites. The factors that may affect the outcome of treatment with the metabolites of D$_3$ include the severity of bone disease and the prevailing plasma level of calcium[10,62], which in turn may reflect the degree of parathyroid autonomy. Patients with high levels of plasma calcium respond poorly and the risks of inducing hypercalcaemia and soft tissue calcification are proportionately greater. The use of these agents, however, does not appear to aggravate vascular or corneal deposits, provided that plasma phosphate is controlled and prolonged hypercalcaemia is avoided. In

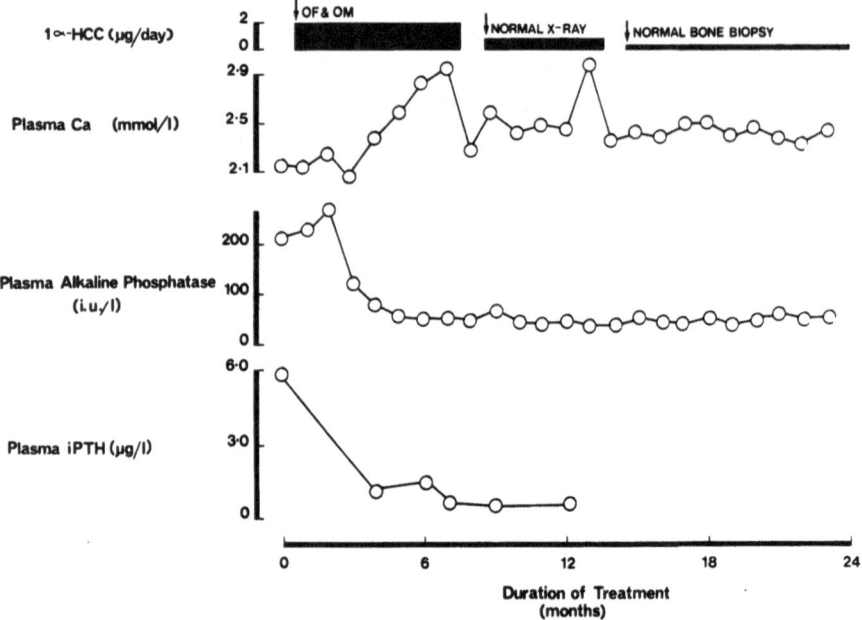

Figure 10.8 Long-term treatment of renal bone disease with lα-hydroxychole-calciferol (1α-HCC) in a dialysis-treated patient with renal bone disease. Healing of osteitis fibrosa (OF) and osteomalacia (OM) occurred within 15 months. Episodes of hypercalcaemia occurred suddenly and the dose of 1α-HCC tolerated decreased when plasma alkaline phosphatase had fallen to normal levels (from Kanis et al.[58])

patients with severe metastatic calcification, parathyroidectomy or transplantation should be considered.

A potential advantage in the use of a metabolite whose production is impaired is that a decreased dose range may be required compared with the parent vitamin. However, in patients with osteitis fibrosa or osteomalacia, the dose needed of 1α-hydroxy metabolites may also change abruptly over an 8-fold range at various stages of treatment[58]. In general, the dose tolerated (in order to avoid hypercalcaemia) decreases with time (Figure 10.8). The greatest risk of hypercalcaemia occurs at the start of treatment and later when biochemical responses are nearing completion[62]. Plasma calcium should be monitored frequently during those risk periods. Currently, there is no evidence that the metabolites of vitamin D exert therapeutic effects in any way different from the parent compound. However, in the case of 1,25-dihydroxycholecalciferol and its synthetic analogue, 1α-hydroxycholecalciferol, their rapid onset and reversal of biological activity confer significant advantages over other preparations

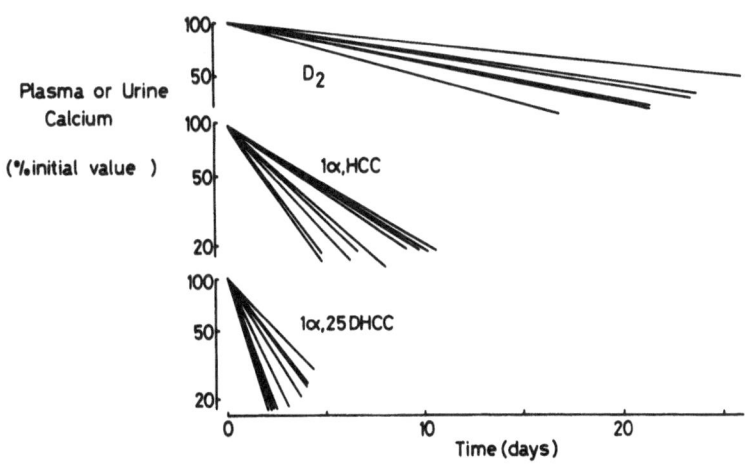

Figure 10.9   Rate of reversal of biological effects after stopping vitamin D₂ and the 1α-hydroxylated derivatives. The fall of plasma or urine calcium (observed minus asymptotic value) is shown on a logarithmic scale and expressed as a percentage of the initial value. (From Kanis and Russell[63])

(Figure 10.9)[63]. The dose may be more easily and rapidly titrated against requirements and inadvertent overdose more rapidly corrected with the 1α-hydroxylated metabolites than with vitamin D_3, D_2, dihydrotachysterol, or 25-hydroxycholecalciferol.

It might be expected that the widespread use of the vitamin D metabolites might eventually decrease the need for parathyroidectomy. At present there is still a need for parathyroidectomy where medical management has failed to improve bone disease or where metastatic calcification and hypercalcaemia are present. In patients with severe bone disease, especially in children where complications may develop rapidly, urgent parathyroidectomy may be considered. However, even in severe and rapidly progressive bone disease, a trial of medical treatment is well worthwhile and serves a dual purpose: if bone disease is rapidly controlled the need for parathyroidectomy may be avoided; if, on the other hand, there remains the need for surgery, the prior treatment with 1α-hydroxylated metabolites of D_3 will considerably decrease the post-operative complications of parathyroidectomy[64] (hypocalcaemia, hungry bones syndrome).

Total parathyroidectomy has been advocated on the grounds that the stimulus for the secretion of parathyroid hormone persists post-operatively and parathyroid hyperplasia will recur[65]. Developments in recent years allow this view to be challenged with increasing confidence. Though parathyroidectomy may be followed by rapid and striking improvements in osteitis fibrosa, pruritis and ectopic calcification[4] (Figure 10.7), patients may be left with persistent osteomalacia, refractory to treatment with vitamin D or its metabolites when total excision is performed. Subtotal parathyroidectomy might also be preferred if the patient is to be transplanted. Finally, if expectations of the ability of the D metabolites to suppress parathyroid gland stimulation are realized by long-term experience, then the use of these metabolites after partial parathyroidectomy may prevent recurrent hyperplasia.

Successful kidney transplantation may rapidly modify renal bone disease. Metastatic calcification and osteitis fibrosa usually regress though healing of bone may take a considerable period of time. Transplantation is, however, associated with an increased incidence of some of the disorders of mineral metabolism, particularly osteopaenia and avascular necrosis[51,53]. Post-transplant hypercalcaemia may give rise to the occasional need for parathyroidectomy[66].

ACKNOWLEDGEMENTS

I am grateful to the Wellcome Trust, the National Kidney Research Fund and the Peel Medical Research Trust for their support in various aspects of this work.

References

1. Avioli, L. V. and Teitelbaum, S. L. (1976). The renal osteodystrophies. In B. M. Brenner and F. C. Rector (eds.). *The Kidney.* pp. 1542–1591. (Philadelphia: W. B. Saunders Company)
2. De Luca, H. F. (1976). Recent advances in our understanding of the vitamin D endocrine system. *J. Lab. Clin. Med.*, **87**, 7
3. Coburn, J. W., Hartenbower, D. L. and Norman, A. W. (1974). Metabolism and action of the hormone vitamin D – Its relation to diseases of calcium homeostasis. *West. J. Med.*, **121**, 22
4. Katz, A. I., Hampers, C. L. and Merrill, J. P. (1969). Secondary hyperparathyroidism and renal osteodystrophy in chronic renal failure. *Medicine*, **48**, 333
5. Kanis, J. A., Adams, N. D., Earnshaw, M., Heynen, G., Ledingham, J. G. G., Russell, R. G. G. and Woods, C. G. (1977). Vitamin D, osteomalacia and chronic renal failure. In A. W. Norman, K. Shaefer, J. W. Coburn, H. F. DeLuca, D. Fraser, H. G. Grigoleit and D. v. Herrath (eds.). *Vitamin D. Biochemical, Chemical and Clinical Aspects Related to Calcium Metabolism.* pp. 671–673. (Berlin: de Gruyter)
6. Kerr, D. N. S., Walls, J., Ellis, D. H., Simpson, W., Uldall, P. R. and Ward, M. K. (1969). Bone disease in patients undergoing regular haemodialysis. *J. Bone Joint Surg.*, **51B**, 587

7. Eastwood, J. B. and De Wardener, H. E. (1975). Renal osteodystrophy. In N. F. Jones (ed.). *Recent Advances in Renal Disease*, 1, 177

8. Mehls, O., Krempien, B., Ritz, E., Scharer, K. and Schuller, H. W. (1973). Renal osteodystrophy in children on maintenance haemodialysis. *Proc. E.D.T.A.*, 10, 197

9. Henderson, R. G., Ledingham, J. G. G. and Woods, C. G. (1974). Renal osteodystrophy in relation to the cause of renal failure. *Kidney Int.*, 6, 62

10. Coburn, J. W., Brickman, A. S., Sherrard, D. J., Singer, F. R., Baylink, D. J., Wong, E. G. C., Massry, S. G. and Norman, A. W. (1977). Clinical efficacy of 1,25-dihydroxy-vitamin D_3 in renal osteodystrophy. In A. W. Norman, K. Shaefer, J. W. Coburn, H. F. DeLuca, D. Fraser, H. G. Grigoleit and D. v. Herrath (eds.). *Vitamin D. Biochemical, Chemical and Clinical Aspects Related to Calcium Metabolism*. pp. 657–666. (Berlin: de Gruyter)

11. Dent, C. E. and Winter, C. S. (1974). Osteomalacia due to phosphate depletion from excessive aluminium hydroxide ingestion. *Br. Med. J.*, 1, 551

12. Rao, T. K. S. and Friedman, E. A. (1975). Fluoride and bone disease in uremia. *Kidney Int.*, 7, 125

13. Slatopolsky, E., Calgar, S., Gradowska, L., Canterbury, J., Reiss, E. and Bricker, N. S. (1972). On the prevention of secondary hyperparathyroidism in experimental chronic renal disease using 'proportional reduction' of dietary phosphorus intake. *Kidney Int.*, 2, 147

14. Bricker, N. S. (1972). On the pathogenesis of the uremic state. *N. Engl. J. Med.*, 286, 1093

15. Reiss, E., Canterbury, J. M. and Kanter, A. (1969). Circulating parathyroid hormone concentration in chronic renal insufficiency. *Arch. Intern. Med.*, 124, 417

16. Coburn, J. W., Popovtzer, M. M., Massry, S. G. and Kleeman, C. R. (1969). The physiochemical state and renal handling of divalent ions in chronic renal failure. *Arch. Intern. Med.*, 124, 302

17. Reiss, E., Canterbury, J. M., Bercovitz, M. A. and Kaplan, E. L. (1970). The role of phosphate in the secretion of parathyroid hormone in man. *J. Clin. Invest.*, 49, 2146

18. Walton, R. J., Russell, R. G. G., Smith, R., Kanis, J. A. and Woodhead, J. S. (1976). The effects of a diphosphonate on phosphate transport in man. In L. Avioli, P. Bordier, H. Fleisch, S. Massry and E. Slatopolsky (eds.). *Phosphate Metabolism, Kidney and Bone*. pp. 329–343. (Toulouse: Nouvelle Imprimerie Fournié)

19. Walton, R. J., Woods, C. G., Russell, R. G. G., Kanis, J. A. and Clark, M. (1976). Histological measurements in Paget's disease of bone and their response to EHDP. *Calc. Tiss. Res.*, 22 (suppl.), 295

20. Bishop, M. C. (1973). Plasma biochemistry in haemodialysed patients. *Lancet*, ii, 1328

21. Baker, L. R. I., Ackrill, P., Cattell, W. R., Stamp, T. C. B. and Watson, L. (1974). Iatrogenic osteomalacia and myopathy due to phosphate depletion. *Br Med. J.*, 3, 150

22. Stanbury, S. W. and Lumb, G. A. (1962). Metabolic studies of renal osteodystrophy. *Medicine*, 41, 1

23. Fraser, D. R. and Kodicek, E. (1970). Unique biosynthesis by kidney of a biologically active vitamin D metabolite. *Nature* (London), 228, 764

24. Mawer, E. B., Backhouse, J., Taylor, C. M., Lumb, G. A. and Stanbury, S. W. (1973). Evidence for failure of formation of 1,25-dihydroxycholecalciferol in chronic renal failure. *Lancet*, i, 626

25. Taylor, C. M. (1977). The measurement of 24,25-dihydroxycholecalciferol in human serum. In A. W. Norman, K. Shaefer, J. W. Coburn, H. F. DeLuca, D. Fraser, H. G. Grigoleit and D. v. Herrath (eds.). *Vitamin D. Biochemical, Chemical and Clinical Aspects Related to Calcium Metabolism.* pp. 541–543. (Berlin: de Gruyter)

26. Kanis, J. A., Heynen, G., Russell, R. G. G., Smith, R., Walton, R. J. and Warner, G. T. (1977). Biological effects of 24,25-dihydroxycholecalciferol in man. In A. W. Norman, K. Shaefer, J. W. Coburn, H. F. DeLuca, D. Fraser, H. G. Grigoleit and D. v. Herrath (eds.). *Vitamin D. Biochemical, chemical and clinical aspects related to calcium metabolism.* pp. 793–795. (Berlin: de Gruyter)

27. Naik, R., Gosling, P., Price, C., Robinson, B. H. B., Dabek, J. T., James, H. M., Kanis, J. A. and Smith, R. (1976). Whole body *in vivo* neutron activation analysis in assessing treatment of renal osteodystrophy with 1α-hydroxycholecalciferol. *Br. Med. J.*, 2, 79

28. Kanis, J. A., Earnshaw, M., Henderson, R. G., Heynen, G., Ledingham, J. G. G., Naik, R., Oliver, D. O., Russell, R. G. G., Smith, R., Wilkinson, R. H. and Woods, C. G. (1977). Correlation of clinical, biochemical and skeletal responses to 1α-hydroxycholecalciferol in renal bone disease. *Clin. Endocrinol.*, 7, 45s

29. DeFronzo, R. A., Andres, R., Edgar, P. and Walker, W. G. (1973). Carbohydrate metabolism in uremia: A review. *Medicine*, 52, 469

30. Gitelman, H. G. (1970). Uremic toxins and mineral metabolism. *Arch. Intern. Med.*, 126, 793

31. Parsons, V., Davies, C., Goode, C., Ogg, C. and Siddiqui, J. (1971). Aluminium in bone from patients with renal failure. *Br. Med. J.*, 4, 273

32. Smith, F. R. and Goodman, D. S. (1971). The effects of disease of the liver and kidneys on the transport of vitamin A in human plasma. *J. Clin. Invest.*, 50, 2426

33. Chertwo, B. S., Williams, G. A., Kiani, R., Stewart, K. L., Hargis, G. K. and Flayter, R. L. (1974). The interactions between vitamin A, vinblastine and cytochalasin B in parathyroid hormone secretion. *Proc. Soc. Exp. Biol. Med.*, 147, 16

34. Feldman, S. L. and Cousins, R. J. (1973). Influence of cadmium on the metabolism of 25-hydroxycholecalciferol in chicks. *Nutr. Rep. Int.*, 8, 4

35. Goodman, A. D., Leman, J., Lennon, E. J. and Relman, A. S. (1965). Production, excretion and net balance of fixed acid in patients with renal acidosis. *J. Clin. Invest.*, 44, 495

36. Pellegrino, E. D. and Biltz, B. S. (1965). The composition of human bone in uremia. *Medicine*, 44, 397

37. MacIntyre, I. (1977). Comparative aspects of the biochemistry of the regulation of vitamin D metabolism. In A. W. Norman, K. Shaefer, J. W. Coburn, H. F. DeLuca, D. Fraser, H. G. Grigoleit and D. v. Herrath (eds.). *Vitamin D. Biochemical, Chemical and Clinical Aspects Related to Calcium Metabolism.* pp. 155–164. (Berlin: de Gruyter)

38. Lancer, S. R., Bowser, E. N., Hargis, G. K. and Williams, G. A. (1976).

The effect of growth hormone on parathyroid function in rats. *Endocrinology*, **98**, 1289

39. Barbour, G. L. and Sevier, B. R. (1974). Adrenal responsiveness in chronic hemodialysis. *N. Engl. J. Med.*, **290**, 1258

40. Heynen, G., Kanis, J. A., Ledingham, J. G. G., Oliver, D. O. and Russell, R. G. G. (1976). Evidence that endogenous calcitonin protects against renal bone disease. *Lancet*, **ii**, 1322

41. Kanis, J. A., Earnshaw, M., Heynen, G., Ledingham, J. G. G., Oliver, D. O., Russell, R. G. G., Woods, C. G., Franchimont, P. and Gaspar, S. (1977). Changes in histologic and biochemical indexes of bone turnover after bilateral nephrectomy in patients on hemodialysis. *N. Engl. J. Med.*, **296**, 1073

42. Parfitt, A. M. (1969). Soft tissue calcification in uremia. *Arch. Intern. Med.*, **124**, 544

43. Mirahmadi, K. S., Duffy, B. S., Shinaberger, J. H., Jowsey, J., Massry, S. G. and Coburn, J. W. (1971). A controlled evaluation of clinical and metabolic effects of dialysate calcium levels during regular hemodialysis. *Trans. Am. Soc. Artif. Intern. Organs*, **17**, 118

44. Henderson, R. G., Kanis, J. A., Ledingham, J. G. G., Oliver, D. O., Russell, R. G. G., Smith, R. and Walton, R. G. G. (1976). Comparative effects of 1α-hydroxycholecalciferol in children and adults with renal glomerular osteodystrophy. In S. P. Nielsen and E. Hjorting-Hansen (eds.). *Calcified Tissues 1975*. pp. 221–225. (Copenhagen: FADL's Forlag)

45. Kanis, J. A., Henderson, R. G., Heynen, G., Ledingham, J. G. G., Russell, R. G. G., Smith, R. and Walton, R. J. (1977). Renal osteodystrophy in non-dialysed adolescents: long-term treatment with 1α-hydroxycholecalciferol. *Arch. Dis. Childh.*, **52**, 473

46. Bishop, M. C., Smith, R., Ledingham, J. G. G. and Oliver, D. O. (1971). Biochemical markers in renal bone disease. *Proc. E.D.T.A.*, **8**, 122

47. Rabinovich, S., Meema, H. E. and Oreopoulos, D. G. (1976). Histological observations of periosteal new bone formation in renal osteodystrophy. In Z. E. G. Zaworski (ed.). *Proceedings of the First Workshop on Histomorphometry*. p. 117. (Ottawa: University Press)

48. Kalu, D. N., Doyle, F. H., Pennock, J. and Foster, G. V. (1970). Parathyroid hormone and experimental osteosclerosis. *Lancet*, **i**, 1363

49. Simpson, W., Ellis, H. A., Kerr, D. N. S., McElroy, M., McNay, R. A. and Peart, K. N. (1976). Bone disease in long-term haemodialysis: the association of radiological with histological abnormalities. *Br. J. Radiol.*, **49**, 105

50. Stanbury, S. W. (1972). Azotemic renal osteodystrophy. In I. MacIntyre (ed.). *Clinics in Endocrinology and Metabolism*. p. 267. (Philadelphia: W. B. Saunders)

51. Atkinson, P. J., Hancock, D. A., Acharya, V. N., Parsons, F. M., Prockor, E. A. and Reed, G. W. (1973). Changes in skeletal mineral in patients on prolonged maintenance dialysis. *Br. Med. J.*, **4**, 519

52. Bone, J. M., Davison, A. M. and Robson, J. S. (1972). Role of dialysate calcium concentration in osteoporosis in patients on haemodialysis. *Lancet*, **i**, 1047

53. Briggs, W. A., Hampers, C. L., Merrill, J. P., Hager, E. B., Wilson, R. E., Birtch, A. G. and Murray, J. E. (1972). Aseptic necrosis in the femur after renal transplantation. *Ann. Surg.*, **175**, 282

54. Ibels, L. S., Stewart, J. H., Mahoney, J. F., Neale, F. C. and Sheil, A. G. R. (1977). Occlusive arterial disease in uraemic and haemodialysis patients and renal transplant recipients. *Q. J. Med.*, **46**, 197

55. Kopple, J. D. and Swendseid, M. E. (1975). Vitamin nutrition in patients undergoing maintenance hemodialysis. *Kidney Int.*, **7**, 79S

56. Sullivan, J. F. and Eisenstein, A. B. (1970). Ascorbic acid depletion in patients undergoing chronic hemodialysis. *Am. J. Clin. Nutr.*, **23**, 1339

57. Eastwood, J. B., Harris, E., Stamp, T. C. B. and DeWardener, H. E. (1976). Vitamin-D deficiency in the osteomalacia of chronic renal failure. *Lancet*, **ii**, 1209

58. Kanis, J. A., Russell, R. G. G. and Smith, R. (1977). Physiological and therapeutic differences between vitamin D, its metabolites and analogues. *Clin. Endocrinol.*, **7**, 191s

59. Clarkson, E. M., Durrant, C., Phillips, M. E., Gower, P. E., Jewkes, R. F. and De Wardener, H. E. (1970). The effect of a high intake of calcium and phosphate in normal subjects and patients with chronic renal failure. *Clin. Sci.*, **39**, 693

60. Goldsmith, R. S., Furszyfer, J., Johnson, W. J., Fournier, A. E. and Arnaud, C. D. (1971). Control of secondary hyperparathyroidism during long term hemodialysis. *Am. J. Med.*, **50**, 692

61. Naik, R. B., Dabek, J. T., Heynen, G., James, H. M., Kanis, J. A., Robertson, P. W., Robinson, B. H. B. and Woods, C. G. (1977). Measurement of whole body calcium in chronic renal failure: effects of 1α-hydroxycholecaciferol and parathyroidectomy. *Clin. Endocrinol.*, **7**, 139s

62. Kanis, J. A., Russell, R. G. G., Naik, R. B., Earnshaw, M., Smith, R., Heynen, G. and Woods, C. G. (1977). Factors influencing the response to 1α-hydroxycholecalciferol in patients with renal bone disease. *Clin. Endocrinol.*, **7**, 51s

63. Kanis, J. A. and Russell, R. G. G. (1977). Rate of reversal of hypercalcaemia and hypercalciuria induced by vitamin D and its 1α-hydroxylated derivatives. *Br. Med. J.*, **1**, 78

64. Boyle, I. T., Fogelman, L., Boyce, B., Thomson, J. E., Beastall, G. H., McIntosh, I. and McLennan, I. (1977). 1α-hydroxy vitamin D_3 in primary hyperparathyroidism. *Clin. Endocrinol.*, **7**, 215s

65. Ogg, C. S. (1967). Total parathyroidectomy in treatment of secondary (renal) hyperparathyroidism. *Br. Med. J.*, **4**, 331

66. Grimelius, L., Johansson, H., Lindquist, B. and Wibell, L. (1972). Tertiary hyperparathyroidism occurring during a renal transplantation programme: report and discussion of three cases. *J. Pathol.*, **108**, 23

DISCUSSION

B. Silke (Dublin): Is there any evidence to suggest that any of the newer analogues are superior to AT 10 in the treatment of renal bone disease?

Cameron: AT 10 is also known as DHT – dihydrotachysterol; it is one preparation of it.

Kanis: There are a number of reports which suggest that there are quite large differences between the various vitamin D-like compounds in their effects upon target tissues. Whether these differences are important in the treatment of renal bone disease is unknown, and there is no convincing evidence, to date, which might suggest that the way in which a therapeutic effect was achieved with one compound differs significantly from the effects of the various other vitamin D-like compounds. However, there is one real advantage in the use of the 1α-hydroxylated metabolites of vitamin D in that their onset and reversal of action is more rapid than that of the other compounds. This means that the dose can be readily titrated according to requirements, and should the patient inadvertently be poisoned, hypercalcaemia may be reversed very rapidly.

Cameron: I can endorse that.

J. S. Robson (Edinburgh): When we think of renal bone disease, we think of the cumulative distortions which have occurred over the previous 5–10 years and there are a number of things that can be unravelled.
    Taking Dr Kanis's three methods of treatment, at what stage should they be applied? What does he think about starting at a very early stage long before there is any clinical evidence, and possibly minimal chemical or bone histological evidence, with the idea of preventing renal bone disease? Would one start before there is any gross architectural distortion that we know to be associated with it?

Kanis: I sympathize with the sentiment that prevention is better than cure. It is certainly possible to modify the natural history of established renal bone disease in some affected patients, but I am not sure whether this use of these agents is pharmacological or physiological, since I am not convinced that the major component of renal bone disease is due to a defective production of 1α-hydroxylated metabolites. Their prophylactic use may not, therefore, be analogous to endocrine replacement therapy.

It is a little early to say with any confidence that renal bone disease could be prevented, although I sympathize with the idea.

Robson: Has anyone tried?

Kanis: A number of trials are currently underway to examine the prophylactic effects of 1,25-dihydroxycholecalciferol and 1α-hydroxycholecalciferol.

R. Ward (Newcastle-upon-Tyne): One of the hallmarks of Newcastle bone disease is that it is unresponsive to D_2, D_3, 1α, 1,25, and DHT, and that it moves on relentlessly.

Has Dr Kanis any comment or experience on this?

Kanis: I hinted briefly that there are large geographical differences in the nature of bone disease seen in various units. 'Newcastle bone disease' is characterized by excessive amounts of osteoid, very few numbers of cells on the osteoid surfaces, and a relatively low level of plasma alkaline phosphatase. It seems to be a kind of osteoblast poisoning which might be due to aluminium, for example in the dialysis fluid or the enthusiastic use of phosphate binders in the past. We do see this type of bone disease, but it occurs in perhaps 2% of our dialysis population and, unlike that of Newcastle, its incidence does not increase with time on dialysis. It is very much more common in Newcastle, but it does occur elsewhere.

F. M. Parsons (Leeds): There is another method by which calcium loss occurs during dialysis, which has been largely ignored. We all know that there is decreased absorption of dietary calcium in renal failure but in addition each time a patient is dialysed about 60 to 100 mg of calcium is removed by ultrafiltration. Further loss occurs when blood is washed back from the dialyser with saline for calcium is not 'reverse dialysed' from dialysate to blood compartment to give a normal diffusible level in the saline. In total a patient can lose anything up to 1700 mg of calcium per week either from the gastrointestinal tract or during dialysis. There will be considerable variation from patient to patient. Some will remain in relatively reasonable calcium balance for they may have better absorption of calcium.

It is all very well talking about the use of vitamin D metabolites or analogues but we must really prevent the negative calcium balance that can be induced by dialysis.

Kanis: Metabolic balance studies are extremely difficult to do on dialysis patients. Dr Bishop in our unit has tried to measure calcium balance in the past, but the techniques used incurred too great an error to provide accurate information.

Parsons: Not the dialysis inaccuracies, surely, for during dialysis there is usually a loss of weight which means that calcium is lost from patient to dialysis fluid.

Kanis: Losses of calcium during dialysis depends on a variety of factors. They depend on the changes in pH, protein concentration and on the duration of dialysis. Perhaps of greatest importance, they depend on the level of calcium that is used in the dialysis fluid. The optimum level of dialysate calcium is not precisely known, but there are data, derived from the rather elegant technique of total body neutron activation analysis, which can give an estimate of calcium balance over a prolonged period of time. The use of dialysate calcium of about 1.65 mmol/l seems to prevent bone loss.

The use of higher concentrations of calcium in the dialysis fluid (up to 2 mmol/l) has been advocated to suppress parathyroid activity but the results are rather disappointing in terms of reversing histologial abnormalities or of decreasing the secretion of parathyroid hormone over the long term. Such procedures also incur the risks of increasing the incidence of metastatic calcification.

We are not neglecting the problem. It is a difficult area to investigate and the successes that have been achieved in that area have been relatively limited.

Cameron: Dr Parsons would like to see the trial with all the regimens that have been mentioned using calcium containing wash-back fluid at the end of the dialysis rather than manipulation of the calcium concentration in the dialysis fluid.

Parsons: As one of the many aspects.

B. H. B. Robinson (Birmingham): Unless one uses excessive volumes, most wash-back fluid does not get into the patient. Most of the blood in the dialyser returns into the patient. I do not think that aspect of technique is very significant in relation to calcium. A few mmols of calcium that will be lost by ultrafiltration will be more than compensated for by using a bath calcium above the level of plasma ultrafilterable calcium. *In vivo* neutron activation studies from our department show that very nearly all patients on dialysis are in positive calcium balance.

Kanis: Various data, using a variety of other techniques, have shown that calcium levels in the dialysis fluid from about 1.63 to 1.75 mmol/l are perhaps the optimum in terms of preventing bone loss and minimizing metastatic calcification.

Parsons: Many other investigations have suggested that it is necessary to have 1.75–2.0 mmol/l of calcium in the dialysis fluid to correct both the ultrafiltration deficit, and also the negative gastrointestinal balance. It is not just the technique of dialysis that leads to a negative balance, but the inability of the intestinal tract to absorb calcium. In fact body calcium is lost into the gastrointestinal tract, and this is where it becomes even more difficult to undertake routine measurements.

Kanis: This is where the technique of whole body *in vivo* neutron activation is ideal, because repeated measurements provide an overall balance measurement. Certainly bone loss during dialysis can be largely prevented.

SECTION FOUR

Psychological and Personal Aspects
Chairman:
M. Carmody

SECTION FOUR

11

Psychological problems of the paediatric haemodialysis patient

D. S. James

11.1   PROBLEMS REFERRED TO IN THE LITERATURE

1.1.1   Mental defence mechanisms

Many papers refer to DENIAL[1-3] which shields a person from facing the severity of his problem and its apparent consequences. In some situations this is an adaptive process, especially in the early stages of a disorder as it may prevent a more serious and complete breakdown. Later it may become maladaptive because if the condition is not accepted, the patient may be prevented from making the right manoeuvres to cope with it. Sand *et al.*[4] say that people do best who discuss their anxieties openly and make no use of mental defence mechanisms which may make them inaccessible to such discussion. Villard[5] found that adults under stress from dialysis polarize into two types. Some become passive and submissive while others over-compensate with optimism or euphoria.

11.1.2   Depression

Abram[6] mentioned four stages of adaptation to dialysis. At first the patient is uraemic, low and depressed for biological reasons. He then begins dialysis and feels an improvement in health but is anxious about the technicalities and fears mechanical failure. In the third stage a reactive depression is likely to occur when the problems of dependency and long-term adaptation to the handicap have to be faced. When this is coped with he enters the fourth phase of rehabilitation. Abram[2] refers to a series of

3478 dialysis patients of whom 166 hastened their death either actively or by passive non-compliance with their treatment regimens.

With children in the early stages of dialysis one finds it difficult to decide to what extent the depressions may be 'biological' and to what extent they are reactive. The mood is sometimes labile on dialysis and can vary markedly from day to day. The use of tricyclic antidepressants in uraemia has been discussed[7] but in children it is often more appropriate to look at ways of adding extra support and helping those caring for the child at home and in hospital to 'tune in' to the patient's distress until the depressive phase passes.

11.1.3 Effects on the family

The spouses of patients undergoing dialysis may require extra support because of the emotional stresses of the situation[8], and in vulnerable families, persons other than the dialysis patient may become mentally ill[9]. A secure marriage not surprisingly suggests that rehabilitation will be successful but unstable marriages may be broken apart. Two papers concerning children undergoing dialysis make similar points. Bernstein[10] reviewed 12 children who were dialysed and then transplanted. Stress symptoms during dialysis often reflected the child's pre-morbid emotional state. The child with previous adjustment problems will find that his maladjustment becomes exacerbated with the added stress of dialysis. The importance of good parental management as a prognostic factor for satisfactory adjustment is also mentioned. Ten of Bernstein's children adapted reasonably well, showing some defences of denial and fantasy, but two broke down with severe depressions and regressive episodes.

Forty-seven children on a dialysis/transplant programme were reviewed from Los Angeles[11] and two distinct problem groups were seen. One group began to withdraw, sleep and turn away and another group became increasingly attention seeking, demanding and dependent. Again the potentiation of family disruption was seen. Where the parents' marriage was vulnerable its break-up was hastened, whereas close caring relationships between the parents caused the family to tighten up into an even more cohesive group.

11.2 THE GLASGOW CHILDREN ON DIALYSIS

11.2.1 Psychiatric assessment

The Renal Unit in the Royal Hospital for Sick Children in Glasgow is just for children. It is an attractive compact ward and communications are good. There have now been 17 children on dialysis aged between 6 and 14 years on arrival. An initial psychiatric interview is done when dialysis is contemplated, along with a psychological assessment giving information about the child's attainments and intelligence. The parents are seen by the psychiatrist to screen them for mental illness and abnormal attitudes, while the psychiatric social worker overlaps and establishes social difficulties and problems in the family pattern of relationships.

11.2.2   The importance of a settled marriage and a settled mother

The data shown in Tables 11.1 and 11.2 is only based on rating scales and opinions, although such soft data sometimes conveys more meaning than more objective tests which may not measure quite what is intended.

Table 11.1 concerns the relationship between psycho-social problems experienced in the family during the child's dialysis and the quality of the parents' marriage rated at the first interview. The marriages were rated on a four point scale: 1. Satisfactory; 2. Stresses contained; 3. Severe stresses and 4. Broken up. In Table 11.1, ratings 1 and 2 are labelled 'marriage satisfactory' and marriages rated 3 or 4 are included under the title 'severe stress or separation'.

TABLE 11.1   Psycho-social problems experienced during dialysis and quality of the parents' marriage at the onset of treatment

	During dialysis	
Marriage at onset	Family cope	Psycho-social problems
Marriage satisfactory	5	0
Severe stress or separation	3	8
Association of problems during dialysis and marital stress before treatment		$P < 0.05$ (Fisher test)

Some of the psycho-social problems encountered included heavy drinking, poor mental health, financial troubles and other manifestations of not coping with the situation.

Although the data is 'soft' there is a significant association between the families that experienced problems during the child's dialysis and those which were under marital stress before the treatment began.

The three misfits in Table 11.1 are all atypical. One family which had

TABLE 11.2   Child's adjustment to dialysis and the mother's mental state at the onset of treatment

Mother's mental state at onset	During dialysis	
	Child copes	Child has symptoms
Mother all right	5	0
Mother; psychiatric problem or mother absent	2	10
Association of child's adjustment problems and impairment of mothering by poor mental health or separation	$P < 0.25$ (Fisher test)	

been separated was reunited, in another, there had been a divorce but the mother was about to remarry, and in the third, a very caring grandmother had taken over.

Table 11.2 is concerned with the relationship between the mother's mental state at the onset of the dialysis and the child's subsequent adjustment to the situation. Although two-thirds of the mothers were rated as showing some impairment, it is not implied that they were sufficiently unwell to merit admission to a psychiatric hospital. These mothers were showing some symptoms of anxiety or depression, were often taking psychotropic drugs and were prone to use the interview situation to discuss their own emotional needs. Where the children had adjustment problems these were likely to be withdrawal, regression, depression or attention demanding. Table 11.2 shows that the child copes best when the mother is in good mental health. The link between neurosis in the mother and symptoms in the child is an important piece of child psychiatry and was highlighted by Professor Rutter in 1966[12].

11.2.3   Intelligence of the children

The measured intelligence quotients ranged from 74 to 142, that is from borderline defective to very bright. Inspection of our data does not yet show intelligence to be related to prognosis for good dialysis. One of our dull children manages very well on home dialysis and the very bright one is doing splendidly as well.

11.2.4   The long-term effects of home dialysis on the family

We have five surviving children who have been on home haemodialysis for several months. In three families the interpersonal relationships are *status quo*. One family shows stress, partly because of social and financial problems resulting from the need to move house and one family has reunited from a previous separation because of the dialysis situation.

11.3 HOW DOES THE FAMILY COPE?

11.3.1 The parental responses

These are some of the ways that enable families to cope with the impact of learning that they have a child with a kidney disorder that will need long-term dialysis. The same principles apply where the child is found to be diabetic, mentally retarded or to be suffering from leukaemia. These reactions are described in textbooks of child psychiatry[13] and are usefully discussed by Steinhauer *et al*.[14].

11.3.1.1 *Denial*

This occurs where the loss of function has not been accepted and if the prognosis is felt to be pessimistic or even incorrect by the parents they may take the child away for another opinion just as treatment is being planned. The same mental mechanism may prevent realistic expectations of the child's limitations and lead to friction between the doctor and the parents. The extent of denial is not a factor of intelligence. Where there is serious illness there is often apparent lack of judgement shown by relatives until they can accept the situation realistically.

11.3.1.2 *Anger*

Sometimes parents will be quite aggressive to medical and nursing staff. This results from a normal grief about the child's loss of function. People can become upset and angry about a fault developing in their car and blame the manufacturer or the garage quite forcibly. The chronic failure of a child's kidney is even more serious and often there is a need to blame someone. Parents may become bitter with their friends but are more likely to find fault with their family doctor or the hospital staff.

11.3.1.3 *Guilt*

Frequently the angry feelings turn inwards as in bereavement reactions and this intra-punitive anger becomes guilt. The parents blame themselves. Perhaps they should have gone to the doctor earlier. Perhaps they should have pushed for a hospital appointment sooner or given better information. 'If only I had not sent him out in the rain and been nicer to him this wouldn't have happened.' Parents may feel to be victims of fate or see the child's disorder as proof of their own inadequacy.

11.3.1.4 *Depression*

If the guilt is not coped with it can precipitate depression and the mood becomes increasingly flat with morbid thoughts, tearfulness and suicidal ideas. Biological symptoms include sleep disturbance, appetite loss and weight changes.

11.3.1.5 *Marital stresses*

Parents faced with a sick child may both want extra emotional support but have little to give. Fathers may escape into working long hours rather than face the demands for support in the home. One parent may adopt a pathological attitude towards the sick child and the other may challenge this with inevitable increasing friction.

11.3.1.6 *The siblings*

Further tension may occur because of the focus onto the sick child who needs to visit the hospital for three days per week. The other children may be somewhat deprived of their usual parental interest but unable to show their displeasure because 'who can be jealous of his sick brother'. The bottled up ill feeling presents in other ways, perhaps as a falling off in school performance, as psychogenic pain or even by joining an antisocial peer group.

11.3.1.7 *Abnormal attitudes*

Although many parents accept the situation and help the child to feel valued, some show *rejection* in various ways. The child may be poorly clad in comparison to his siblings or there may be repeated requests for re-admissions to hospital. A more subtle kind of rejection is shown by parents who initially give the impression that they are very caring. During successive interviews it is noticed that they are dissatisfied with the child's achievements and medical progress, which causes the child to be undermined. They are trying to say 'look what good parents we are, we are doing everything to get him right and still he won't be well'. This is a rejecting attitude masked by an apparent overprotection. The more straightforward *overprotection* is also damaging to the child and occurs where the parents are excessively anxious.

11.3.2   The child's responses

11.3.2.1   *Denial*

As previously mentioned, this mechanism enables the child to exclude stressful situations from his thoughts. The resulting behaviour may appear detached and inconsistent towards the demands of treatment, for example, refusal of a diet which he feels to be unnecessary.

11.3.2.2   *Reaction formation*

This is shown by the child who needs to appear tough and to dominate his friends. From under this defence, frequently emerges a child who is anxious, brittle and eventually discloses a poor self-opinion. A disability requiring dependence on repeated medical treatment is prone to generate this response.

11.3.2.3   *Regression*

This is shown by many children under stress when they become more dependent and infantile. They may crave undivided adult attention, wish to be fed, request medications and make heavy demands on nursing staff.

11.3.2.4   *Obsessions*

Some children indulge in magical thinking. 'If I tap the medicine three times it won't go wrong.' The resulting rituals and unnecessary attention to irrelevant detail may irritate the nursing staff and exhaust the child.

11.3.2.5   *Fantasy*

Younger children may shut out the unpleasant reality world by becoming lost in the more acceptable world of make believe. Much of children's literature and media programmes assume high levels of fantasy.

The above are 'coping mechanisms' which enable the child to remain in reasonable mental health. Where these mechanisms give inadequate protection or where the stresses become too severe the child may break down into illness needing more specialized psychiatric help. The common illnesses are:

11.3.2.6 *Massive withdrawal*

Occurs with blatant lack of cooperation and motivation. A child has been observed where his dialyser became disconnected and he made no effort to raise alarm as the blood poured onto the floor.

11.3.2.7 *Anxiety neurosis*

This may occur with obsessional thinking, feelings of impending doom, tension symptoms and inability to cope.

11.3.2.8 *Depression*

This is also seen with psychogenic pain, sleep disturbance, anorexia, poor concentration, fears and morbid guilty thoughts. Depressed children are clingy to parents and staff and the cheerful approach often lacks empathy and hence fails to alleviate the distress. Much of the above maladaptive behaviour can be averted by attention to the following points.

11.4 HOW TO AVERT PSYCHOLOGICAL PROBLEMS

The emotional impact of a child on long-term dialysis *effects the whole family* either directly or indirectly through the reaction of another family member.

It takes time for those involved to work through the defences and reach a *realistic acceptance* of the situation. The nephrologist should share the details and prognosis with parents at an early stage and enable further discussion time to clarify points which have not been heard (denial) and also show that there are no ill feelings from the parents' initial responses which may have been anger.

Marital stress can be minimized by *seeing both parents together* so that the information is not moulded into armaments for disagreements. *Frequent appointments* should be offered where pathological attitudes develop and the handling of these situations may be passed to an experienced social worker.

Children on dialysis should be encouraged to talk out their fantasy. The conspiracy of silence should be avoided. Children may have gross misconceptions about their kidneys or the dialysis. One child thought he had to go inside the machine to have his blood washed.

The child's *school attainments* should be monitored. Much time can be lost before dialysis and from days off attending the unit. The child feels lost and can 'give up'. Our own unit has a teacher and the education authorities can usually provide extra help if the problem is made clear to them. These children will rely on non-physical jobs when they grow into adult life and education is especially important. Staff working in renal units should *not bear hostility personally*. Reasons for parental anger and non-cooperation from children have been discussed. To turn against one's clients in confrontation will play into the psychopathology.

The team approach can be helpful in dealing with psycho-social problems and community links including the child's school. Regular case conferences involving nephrologist, nurses, dietician, teacher, play leader, social worker, psychologist and psychiatrist can ensure good communications between those involved. The team should not however encroach on the medical management decisions and the team leader should be the nephrologist in charge.

Nursing staff should not rival with the parents. The dependency of the child meets a vocational emotional need in a caring nurse. Parents may resent the child's attachment to nursing staff and it is easy to undermine a parent with social problems, which may increase the child's distress and cause the family to find fault with the unit. Nevertheless the nurse or doctor will get to know the dialysis children intimately, and like the good parent, they *must set limits* on the child's behaviour. It is caring to enforce diet, treatment and reasonable conduct but this should be done with a positive relationship so that the patient does not feel disliked. It is this trusting relationship that is the major defence against the emergence of psychopathology.

References

1. Glassman, B. M. and Siegel, A. (1970). Personality correlates of survival in a long-term hemodialysis program. *Arch. Gen. Psychiat.*, **22**, 566
2. Abram, H. S. (1970). Survival by machine: the psychological stress of chronic hemodialysis. *Psychiat. Med.*, **1**, 37
3. Short, M. J. and Wilson, W. P. (1969). Roles of denial in chronic hemo-dialysis. *Arch. Gen. Psychiat.*, **20**, 433
4. Sand, P., Livingston, G. and Wright, R. G. (1966). Psychological assessment of candidates for a hemodialysis program. *Ann. Intern. Med.*, **64**, 602
5. Villard, H. P. (1969). The psychiatric consultant in the renal dialysis and transplant unit. *Un. Med. Canada*, **98**, 233
6. Abram, H. S. (1969). The psychiatrist, the treatment of chronic renal failure and the prolongation of life. *Am. J. Psychiat.*, **126**, 157
7. Neary, D. (1976). Neuropsychiatric sequelae of renal failure. *Br. J. Hosp. Med.*, **15**, 122
8. Shambaugh, P. W. and Kanter, S. S. (1969). Spouses under stress: group meetings with spouses of patients on hemodialysis. *Am. J. Psychiat.*, **125**, 928

9. Cramond, W. A. (1971). Renal transplantations – experiences with recipients and donors. *Sem. Psychiat.*, 3, 116
10. Bernstein, D. M. (1970). Emotional reactions of children and adolescents to renal transplantation. *Chld. Psychiat. Hum. Devel.*, 1, 102
11. Korsch, B. M., Fine, R. N., Grushkin, C. M. and Negrete, V. F. (1971). Experiences with children and their families during extended hemodialysis and kidney transplantation. *Pediat. Clin. N. Am.*, 18, 625
12. Rutter, M. (1966). Children of sick parents; an environmental and psychiatric study. *Maudsley Monogr. no. 16.* Oxford University Press
13. Kanner, L. (1957) *Child Psychiatry*, 3rd edn. (Springfield, Ill.: Charles C. Thomas)
14. Steinhauer, P. D., Mushin, D. N. and Rae-Grant, Q. (1974). Psychological aspects of chronic illness. *Pediat. Clin. N. Am.*, 21, 825

12

Social and psychological problems of the adult haemodialysis patient
Kirsty M. Marshall and
T. Walmsley

12.1 INTRODUCTION

In this paper we will describe the process of adjustment to treatment on dialysis, giving some attention to significant problems of adaptation, with examples. Chronic illness is recognized to be a family problem, and we will describe briefly some of the family demands and adjustments which are necessary for successful dialysis; and we shall discuss the importance of inter-disciplinary involvement in helping patients with the psycho-social problems of their treatment.

12.2 THE PATIENT

12.2.1 Emotional stresses

It has long been recognized that patients on chronic dialysis are faced with a variety of emotional stresses as a result of their illness and treatment.[1] Briefly, some of these problems are: fear of dying, and of frequent subjections to pain and illness; fear of loss of job and income; uncertainty about the future; changes in life-style, family and social status.

The most important step in assessing the patient's eventual response to the onset of renal failure is to observe his reaction to the illness in its initial stages. The degree of acceptance which each person and his family achieves dictates much to his ultimate well-being and successful adaptation.

12.2.2 Grief reaction

It is usual for people to approach severe physical loss through a process of realization which is akin to grief.[2] 'The reaction to loss of a limb, and for that matter to loss of function of a vital part is grief and depression'[3]. The patient moves from denial of the loss towards a gradual acceptance. Patients who have been told of the nature and severity of their illness may deny the information, even when this has been most carefully and explicitly shared. Such denial is a mechanism for coping with initial shock and for avoiding overwhelming anxiety and seems to be necessary for many people before the full implication of the illness can be recognized.

12.2.3 Anxiety

As realization dawns, denial may be replaced by acute anxiety, when the patient comes to depend very heavily on the support and understanding of hospital staff, and needs the comfort of relatives and friends. Reassurance is inadequate at this stage. It is important that the patient should be helped to express feelings of anxiety which assist him in moving towards greater self-assertiveness.

It is well established that many patients become preoccupied with events leading up to the onset of illness which is paralleled by the 'regret' of bereavement. Some patients single out particular events which, to them, appear significant, even if apparently unrelated to the disease. A patient told us in all seriousness that his health had begun to deteriorate following an accident at work. He was a railwayman who some years before becoming ill had his foot crushed by a train. He was convinced that his renal failure in some way was provoked by this event.

Anger may be directed towards doctors or other people who could have prevented the onset of illness and the patient may bitterly regret some action of his own. Some patients fail to move beyond the stage of feeling bitter and angry about the injustice of illness. This is wasteful of the emotional energy which should be directed towards effective rehabilitation. One patient, a miner, spent all his dialysis life 'fighting for his cause' in bitter recriminations against doctors and his local community to the extent that he was quite unable to return to any kind of positive existence at home or at work.

12.2.4 Sexual problems

Concern about 'loss of self' or mutilation is paramount for most patients, fears of 'never being the same again', of being changed and damaged. Such feelings reflect the importance of self-image and maintenance of self-esteem. Sexual problems are probably related to interference with body-image, and patterns of sexual functioning amongst renal patients are very variable. Some patients remain sexually active, despite other physical limitations from the illness, while others may be impotent. Potency seems to relate more to emotional well-being and self-esteem than to the degree of physical disability. Here too, it is important to examine pre-dialysis behaviour. A man who had considerable dependency needs and always 'enjoyed ill health', was described by his wife as having 'everything he ever wanted' once he started dialysis, whilst another, who was previously very concerned with schemes for improving his physical fitness, was unable to tolerate what seemed like the personal and physical assault of renal failure.

12.2.5 Importance of assessment

In establishing a programme of support for dialysis patients and their families, it has been useful to recognize the similarities with the process of bereavement. It is possible to identify and prevent reactions which complicate progress towards healthy adaptation. Difficulties arise from distortion of this process, from unresolved anger and depression. Dependent patients may find the life-supporting equipment terrifying and lapse into an attitude of helpless invalidism. Over-assertive patients may adopt a defence of denial which collapses catastrophically later in treatment. A depressive state frequently centres on ruminations of loss; loss of kidney function, of health and well-being, of previous occupational and social adjustment.

12.2.6 Symptoms of stress

During the training phase of treatment, psychiatric problems may be manifest as non-verbal cues. Lateness in arrival for hospital dialysis, difficulties in cannulation, refusal to look at the dialysis machine and an increase in non-specific symptoms may mark unspoken ambiguities of feeling towards the continuation of treatment. Occasionally frank neurotic states such as phobias or dissociation may supervene in the patient or his spouse. The patient on home dialysis may feel deserted by the hospital team and behave with hostility or indifference at out-patient attendances. Dialysis may become irregular and be accompanied by manipulative and attention-seeking behaviour. Repeated admissions with metabolic embarrassment or dietary indiscretion and associated weight gain are often the hallmark of such patients with separation anxiety. Here, the family around the patient is of key importance.

12.3 THE FAMILY

Successful dialysis depends on the support of the family, and its members may experience considerable stress in coping with treatment over a protracted period of time. Much depends on established patterns of family and marital behaviour prior to the onset of treatment. The continuous crisis of regular dialysis may lead to polarization of behaviour, sometimes aggravating an existing family problem, although previously poor relationships may sometimes be improved. For example, a patient whose renal failure had developed insidiously over some years, had severe marital problems by the time she was referred for treatment. It was an immense relief to both her and her husband to discover another explanation for her behaviour, and the shared experience of home dialysis was constructive in re-establishing a positive relationship.

  The unrelenting nature of the illness and constant climate of uncertainty is difficult for many couples, who describe the need to readjust their values in learning to live from day to day and to limit expectations for the future. This can be positive as well as negative, but attitudes depend on individual aspirations and achievements. An older patient who is married and a father has valued the extra life granted to him by dialysis and can enjoy, at secondhand, the accomplishments of his children. A young single man has limited investment in dialysis because of curtailed opportunities for fulfilling hopes and ambitions.

Every family is faced by the challenge of adjustment. It is not only that the machine makes extra demands, but that responsibilities are shared differently. So much energy goes into maintaining basic tasks of living and working that other matters assume lower priority. This may include management of the children as well as decision making and financial responsibilities. It seems that where the whole family can be involved in recognizing and accepting the changes which are inevitable – where children, for example, can be helped to contribute in a positive way to the family's tasks – the effect can be to unify all the members.

For some families the demands of dialysis have been met by quite major role changes. These may be reasonable and healthy for particular family needs, even if bizarre to others. It is important to assess each individual family's functioning, and to help the members to achieve their own answers for coming to terms with dialysis treatment. This demands a high level of understanding of individual needs and difficulties by all members of the care team.

12.4 TEAM MEETINGS

Experience in the Medical Renal Unit in Edinburgh suggests that considerable morbidity in chronic patients can be avoided by the institution of regular team meetings. These occur weekly and last 1 hour. Face-to-face contact is regarded as essential and there is no agenda. All team members are encouraged to bring up any contemporary difficulties in patient management. As the meetings proceed such difficulties frequently bring to light differences in staff attitudes which can be squarely faced. Confrontation in the presence of a disinterested third party frequently permits a reformulation and resolution of the difficulty. There is a clear conclusion here: patient morbidity often reflects conflict among the staff. Some staff may be over-protective of a particular patient while others are covertly rejecting[4]. Bringing such a difference to the surface improves the care of the patient and increases the cohesiveness of the unit staff.

12.5 CONCLUSION

Chronic dialysis is usefully regarded as a non-specific stress to which certain personalities are peculiarly vulnerable. At the inception of treatment, anxiety should be regarded as the norm. Terror, hostility or bland acceptance may signal chronic psychological instability and require psychiatric exploration. The main bulk of psychiatric morbidity in dialysis patients consists of neurotic illness and the reactions of abnormal personalities. Acute confusional states and transient paranoid psychoses are occasional hazards of treatment; chronic organic psychosis is rare.

In the care of the patient on chronic haemodialysis two groups are usually involved. The patient's family have to make considerable adjustment and often require professional help to do so. The dialysis team is a second group which often reflects the conflicts of the first and which by deliberate recognition of its psycho-social problems can better serve its patients and increase its future effectiveness.

References

1. Cramond, W. A., Knight, P. R. and Lawrence, J. R. The psychiatric contribution to a renal unit undertaking chronic haemodialysis and renal homotransplantation. *Br. J. Psychiat.*, 113, 1201
2. Parkes, C. M. (1972). *Bereavement: Studies of Grief in Adult Life.* (London: Tavistock Publications)
3. Fisher, S. H. (1960). Psychiatric conditions of hand disability. *Arch. Phys. Med. Rehab.*, 41, 62
4. Kaplan De-Nour, A. and Czaczkes, J. W. (1968). Emotional problems and reactions of the medical team in a chronic haemodialysis unit. *Lancet*, ii, 987

DISCUSSION

Miss H. Rosenthal (London): Has either of the speakers any experience of working with groups of dialysis patients?

Miss K. M. Marshall: Not groups of patients, but we do have a spouse group in Edinburgh which has been running for almost 4 years. Patients sometimes reject that kind of contact with each other. In Edinburgh they will meet informally in the unit, but they have often avoided any other kind of contact. Individual patients have tried to institute this, but it has not been successful.

The spouse group have given each other a tremendous amount of support and they have been able to acknowledge some of their fears, fears about death of the partner and so on, quite directly with each other.

D. S. James (Glasgow): We have purposefully had no group for the children. There is a big scatter of age and intelligence. Some patients are at a much more advanced stage of understanding and coping with the mechanisms than others, and a group would not gel.

In addition to that, most of the patients come into the unit for 3 days a week, and if they were to get together in a group a number of them would have to come in for an extra day. Ours is a regional centre and some of them come a long way and they would not want to come another day.

We have been talking about a parent group. We feel that it is something we should perhaps venture to establish, and now that the unit has been running for 4 years it is probably time we did something about it.

A. L. G. Moss (Nottingham): May I endorse what Miss Marshall said about groups. In our own unit we have experimented with a group for spouses. At the beginning we did think about providing something for the patients, but we decided that the real need wasn't there, it was for the spouses, and that was borne out by the work we have done with them since. If it can be accomplished, then I would recommend that way of working for renal units. The same must go for parents of child patients. The spin-offs are fantastic. The kind of inter-reaction achieved in that type of group situation in terms of mutual support and people being able to air what they really feel about things is much greater than would be achieved on an individual one-to-one basis. A further benefit that we have had has been a patients' association which grew from the first of our groups and which has been able to make a large contribution to the work of the unit in the City.

Mrs J. A. Lipman (London): If there is no children's group as such, how do the children react within the unit?

James: The children on dialysis are usually in separate cubicles, which reduces the amount of contact. There is one room where two children are dialysed together, and usually the television is on, although there are pairs that communicate fairly openly with each other.

We have a play leader and a teacher, and in term time there is one-to-one assistance going for a bit of the time where they would otherwise be interacting.

I am sure that there is a lot of informal contact, but there is no great fostering of a group feeling.

A. Murphy (Glasgow): In general, contact is good, but it has positive and negative effects. The child who is self-cannulating can produce a positive or a negative effect on the non-cannulating child opposite. By and large we feel that it is good to keep the children together and in contact. In our situation two are in contact and one is on his own and we move them around. The children get on well with each other. Outside the hospital they are beginning to see each other socially.

Mackenzie (Canada): Our diagnostic guidelines are probably at an adequate stage to recommend that just as a particular physical finding, e.g. blood pressure, is monitored regularly, we could monitor psychological dimensions. For example, the degree of denial, the amount of regression, the amount of assumption of personal control over dialysis events, and so on. Perhaps it would be useful to think of including as a regular monitoring dimension psychological attributes along with physiological ones. That would help to sharpen up our application of sometimes woolly behavioural ideas, particularly for staff who are not particularly trained in psychiatric terminology.

Miss Marshall mentioned impotence as being a fairly common problem. In my own experience in our unit there is often a general diminution of interest in sexual function during a dialysis period, but in a number of patients, probably one third to one half – and I believe that this is reflected in other units – after transplant impotence becomes a major problem. This seems to be regardless of physiological findings and it is certainly not related to other evidence of peripheral neuropathy, and it presumably has a psychological component. Many of the cases I have seen have otherwise seemed to have quite satisfactory psychological adaptations, and I am at a bit of a loss to explain the discrepancy. Perhaps there is some symbolic significance of having a foreign object in the pelvic area. I do not know the reason, but the experience is shared in other units.

James: On the question of whether to monitor the mental mechanisms in a more systematic way, we re-assess our children from time to time but I have some misgivings about it. I do not know that too much intrusion of psychiatry and psychology in the formal way of testing is particularly helpful to people who already have a damaged self-esteem. One would hope that if a unit is functioning properly – and I think that I can say this of the Glasgow unit – that the nursing staff, the dietician, the play leader and the nephrologist are sufficiently in contact to be able to monitor these things almost intuitively, which in many ways is a better measure than a test.

In any case, although I have shown that there are marital problems and difficulties in families with coping and that some of the children throw off some of these defence mechanisms, at the end of the day I am not sure. The children on home dialysis still have their dialysis irrespective of these factors. If I had been allowed my head, then the first two children, who are fairly successfully managing at home, would have been over-protected and not allowed that chance, because I would have said that it was too difficult. The medical and paediatric approach which optimistically assumes that they will cope has paid off. I must therefore have some anxieties about how intrusive the psychiatrist becomes.

Mackenzie: If I might respond to that. We routinely use problem-oriented records and I can see nothing wrong with self-care, for example, or ability to learn, as being an item on a problem list.

C. Burdett (Leicester): We have heard something of the problem of stress resulting in a person becoming less able to cope with the situation. I would suggest that a model of the person under stress is the person on the machine. I would also suggest that the various defence mechanisms are merely reflections of stimulus avoidance. We should be working towards diminishing fear response by graded exposures of the patients towards the fear.

James: Modelling is very important. There are two principles involved in the interactions between parents and their children. The behavioural approach with the consistency of reward and punishment, modelling and learning is one. The other has to do with the more analytical approach and the relationship between the two.

When dealing with neuroses in childhood, the parent becomes depressed and the child no longer has his needs provided. The mother becomes irascible, complains of being made ill, of being given a headache. She tells the child to go away and that they cannot go out. At other times she will feel guilty because she is depressed and she will try to make up to the child. This is clearly seen in the school phobic situation where the mother will lose her temper one day because the doctor says the child is all right. Then the next day she will be all over him because he has been sent home from school. She feels she is a bad mother, and wonders if the child is all right. Given this subtle sharing of a neurosis which usually begins with the parent and then involves the child, the modelling explanation is much too simple, and in these situations we are seeing both principles. If there is a long-standing conduct disorder, or a personality disorder, then modelling is very important. If it is a middle-class well-put-together biddable over-protective family, then sometimes the analytical or psychotherapy model may get one further in putting in the necessary corrective counselling.

13

Haemodialysis – a personal viewpoint
J. C. Baillie

I developed a renal problem in December 1973 and I spent most of 1974 on an in-patient and out-patient basis at the Royal Infirmary of Edinburgh.

My introduction to the 'Kidney Machine' is rather hazy as I was very ill at the time and I did not appreciate the gravity of the situation. When I did realize what was happening to me I was very frightened and insecure.

In due course I was discharged from hospital and attended the Medical Renal Unit twice a week for dialysis. These were 10-hour sessions every Wednesday and Sunday. I was often unwell during and after dialysis. The next day was also often uncomfortable, with stomach cramp and sickness.

It was about this time that I realized this was to be a permanent situation and if I were to stay alive I would have to learn to live with it. I went through a period of depression when problems seemed insurmountable and coping with life was difficult and tiresome. I·dreaded the hospital dialysis days and was thankful that there were only two per week.

The staff in the Medical Renal Unit began to educate me in the basic principles of dialysis and in the necessary physiological adaptations which would be required for this procedure to work.

As an in-patient I had a Teflon shunt implanted in my leg, providing a connection for the machine. This first shunt and a subsequent one in the other leg proved unsatisfactory for long-term dialysis and I had to undergo another minor operation so that a permanent Cimino fistula could be constructed in my arm. This ensured entry and exit points for the blood during dialysis. This part of haemodialysis is still an unpleasant operation, as a needle wrongly placed can cause a blood flow problem and running repairs are necessary.

I now had to consider returning to business and was greatly helped by a sympathetic company who were most helpful in adjusting my gradual return to work. At this time I occasionally felt unwell and often collapsed, even in the street. I made a concentrated effort to play a useful and profitable part in the commercial world again and I think that this, along with quiet encouragement from my family, helped me to accept the situation in which I found myself.

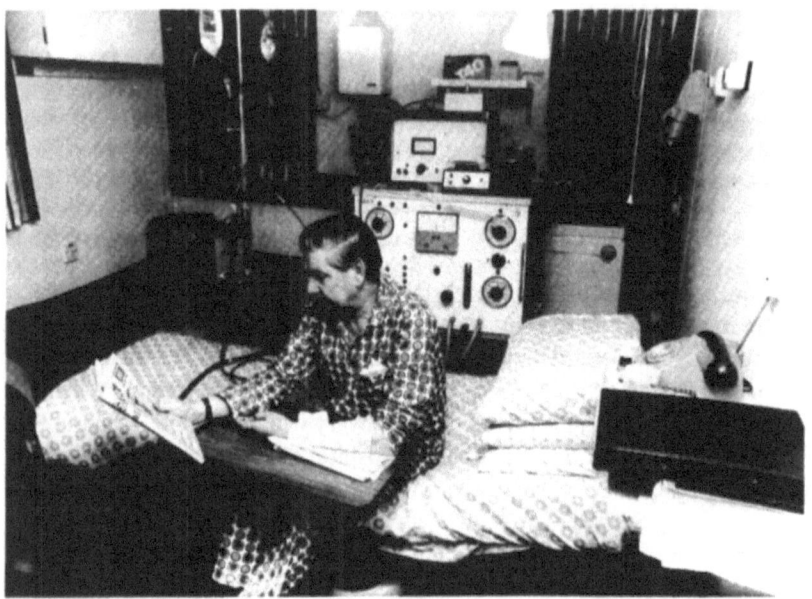

Figure 13.1   Interior of Portakabin

Regular dialysis and a strict low sodium diet slowly improved my health. The lack of salt in food makes the diet boring and tasteless, but I firmly believe that adhering to the diet makes the difference between being well and unwell (although I would never admit this to my dietitian). Compensation is round the corner, as I can have a meal of my choice while dialysing. Fluid intake is limited to 600 ml per day and my party piece about this is that if I am only allowed 600 ml of fluid a day, I would rather have it as whisky!

Once it had been proved that I was a successful dialysis patient, home dialysis was suggested to me. Treatment three times a week would be beneficial and I had the necessary facilities in my garden for a Portakabin. I also had an attendant, my wife, to help operate and maintain the Portakabin and its contents. Home dialysis appealed to my wife and myself from the start. Hospital dialysis had been a very time-consuming operation, involving 10–12 hours per treatment and often terminating at 2 or 3 o'clock in the morning. After this I had to drive home feeling unwell and unable to sleep. Also, we hoped to make a routine which would least affect the family and my work.

Just over a year after I had my first dialysis, a Portakabin was placed in my garden by the local authority and the necessary equipment was installed. This placed the responsibility of working the machine with my wife and myself. It was with some apprehension that we prepared for our first dialysis, but a nurse from the Medical Renal Unit guided us through our first week. Then we were on our own. An efficient back-up service of technicians and administrators were, however, only a 'phone call' away.

Even at home, dialysis is still a time-consuming operation. Dialysing for 6 hours three times a week and preparing the machine, etc. I spend 27 hours a week in the Portakabin. In addition to this, my wife has to clean the floor and all surfaces after each dialysis. Businesswise, I have the same problem – time. I should be more mobile in my job than I am, although I did manage a quick trip to Finland last autumn.

Home dialysis has improved my health immensely and the benefit of dialysing three times a week has become apparent as I have returned to my normal weight and to a feeling of physical well-being. In general, I find that I can cope much better with life. The machine is no longer the MONSTER it was and the unit is now referrred to by the family as 'THE SLAMMER'. Holidays are a big problem as far as the family are concerned and I miss my 3 weeks' fishing holiday in the Western Highlands in the summer.

A kidney transplant, I suppose, has always been in my mind, but I realize that as a successful dialysis patient I am a low priority for transplantation. If I were offered a transplant I would have to consider it very carefully, as I now keep in very good health and I know that my machine will not reject. It may hiccup occasionally, but that is all.

So what have we got to look forward to? We look forward to new and improved equipment which will cut down dialysis time and perhaps to the use of a mobile unit for holidays and perhaps to a MIRACLE.

14

Haemodialysis and transplantation – a personal experience
J. A. Henry

A previous speaker at this symposium gave us food for thought when he posed the question, 'how meaningful is this life?'. And he gave us an answer when he told us that not one of 350 patients, once given a trial of haemodialysis, refused to continue. Each case history represents the story of an individual and his will to live.

Very often the doctor can only attempt a guess at the real feelings and the difficulties that his patient is experiencing. As a doctor who has been through chronic renal failure, 7 years of haemodialysis and a renal transplant, I would like to comment on some aspects of the experience I have undergone. After 8 years of chronic glomerulonephritis from 1961 to 1969, I was started on home haemodialysis following 2 months of hospital dialysis. At that time I dialysed on my own for three 10-hour sessions each week. Life on haemodialysis was often not easy, but I managed to stay at work regularly and to fulfil the long hours demanded of a house physician. In the beginning I was so pleased to be alive and able to work that I did not seriously consider renal transplantation.

Once a patient is established on haemodialysis the prognosis is good, But the really long-term figures, of the order of 10 years, are still insufficient to draw reliable conclusions, particularly as many of the patients who form the basis for these figures were among the very first patients to be dialysed. I think I could be considered as one of the 'second generation' of haemodialysis patients – I was not moribund at the start, I was on home haemodialysis, my blood pressure was always well controlled and I was never transfused for chronic anaemia. Consequently, I viewed my prognosis on haemodialysis as excellent.

Many informed and educated patients once established on haemodialysis are very reluctant to put their names forward for transplantation, because of the risk it represents, even though it may liberate them from all the difficulties that accompany dialysis. Spending about 30 hours per week preparing, or being attached to, or clearing up after using a kidney machine, is a big limitation. On top of that are the restrictions in diet and fluid intake with the social difficulties entailed. Chronic tiredness, job difficulties, family tensions, dependence on a machine, and many other aspects of the enforced change in lifestyle makes dialysis an experience which requires considerable adaptation and a lot of effort.

Being a doctor made it even more difficult for me in the beginning, because I understood all the risks and complications of the various aspects of my treatment right from the start. Later on, I think it became an advantage, because I was able to manage my health more carefully. My relationships with the medical staff in charge of my case were always good. I often had strong ideas about my management and put my case forcibly at times but I always followed their advice faithfully. On only one occasion – which I shall mention later – did I deliberately mislead them.

In the background, however, was the constant dream of leading a dialysis-free life. I longed for a way of life away from the stresses of dialysis, from which there is no break, no holiday. And the only way to this was through a renal transplant. I knew the risks; the main ones that concerned me were the mortality, together with the morbidity – from the operation, with all its technical complications, and also from rejection, infection, malignant disease and osteoporosis. Cadaver transplantation has a mortality of around 25% over the first 2 years, with a further 25% of patients returning to dialysis. The figures improve considerably with a living related donor, and are probably better if the patient is healthy and managing well on dialysis, but they remain daunting. I have several friends who intend to remain on dialysis because they do not see transplantation as an acceptable alternative[1]. The gamble of a one in four mortality is not lightly undertaken, particularly when there is no guarantee for the survivor that his quality of life will necessarily be better after transplantation.

An acid test is to ask the people who know all the arguments. I have made a point of asking a number of nephrologists the telling question, 'Would you, if you were established on dialysis, choose to have a renal transplant?' The invariable answer is 'I would stay on dialysis'. These same doctors recommend renal transplantation to their patients. I can perfectly understand their attitude; by offering transplantation they are able to do more good to more patients with the available resources. Their moral dilemma is a very real one. Dialysis, apart from being a far from ideal treatment, is a luxury that cannot be provided in an unlimited way, although it undoubtedly offers the best chance of survival. The ideal solution is to have a functioning transplant without the hazards of conventional immunosuppressive therapy, but that is clearly a long way off.

At the time, I never really considered the ethics of my initial refusal to be transplanted, or whether other patients were being denied a place on a dialysis programme because of it. Looking back, I believe from an ethical standpoint that individual freedom takes precedence in these matters.

For $4\frac{1}{2}$ years I refused even to allow my blood to be taken for tissue typing. I was keeping reasonably well and was pushing ahead with a career in hospital medicine. Transplantation is an open-ended commitment; with all its uncertainties and its considerable morbidity I might no longer be able to plan my life or to remain at work so predictably.

However, as time went on, I gave more and more serious consideration to transplantation, and added weight was given to my thoughts by the occurrence of painful Looser's zones in my ribs and stress fractures of the metatarsals due to prolonged therapy with aluminium hydroxide. However, it had its desired effect, because there was no trace of ectopic calcification after 7 years on dialysis, and in fact the bony complications all healed rapidly with reduction in the dose of aluminium hydroxide.

In 1974, I was attending hospital for a routine check, when a technician came to take blood for tissue typing. I let her go ahead. If I had been asked in advance, I think I would have refused. The result was then entered in the computer system of the National Organ Matching and Distribution Service. This provoked further thoughts on transplantation, and I began to think about a living related donor kidney. I had my blood tissue typed at a hospital other than my own. The result was stuck on the wall of my dialysis room for several months before I took any action. Eventually I asked my parents to be tissue typed. Both had acceptable ABO groups and each had two out of four antigens. Both my sisters were also tissue typed. Neither of them was HLA identical; they were both quite disappointed.

I was still slowly pondering the problem, but taking no positive steps, till just a year ago, when my arm was forced by a telephone call which said, 'HLA identical kidney for you in Liverpool'. A four antigen – 'full house' –

match is too rare an opportunity to refuse. Any misgivings were thrown overboard, and I fell for the bait with a sense of elation. If it had been anything less than identical I do not think I would have accepted it. I went immediately to the hospital and had the necessary x-rays and microbiological investigations. I dialysed that night. The following day I went to hospital to work as usual; the promise of a transplant was not yet confirmed. However, during the day I had a cryptic message telling me to 'starve'. I knew what it meant and went to hospital for the operation.

The first week after transplantation is still very hazy. I was told afterwards of a number of visitors that I had spoken to, but I have no recollection to this day of their having visited me. I do remember my fascinated delight at seeing *my* urine collecting in a bag by the bedside, having been produced by someone else's kidney. The intensive care, with monitor and intravenous infusions, I took very much for granted. The pain was considerable, bladder spasms were trying and the wound was quite sore, but I was able to sit up and walk quite quickly.

My first excursion outside the hospital was 9 days after the operation, and I left the hospital for lunch with friends on the 10th day. By the 11th day I considered my rehabilitation complete when I went to a local hostelry for a pint of beer. I remember my surpise when I felt the call of nature and had to ask the way to the convenience. I had had many gin-and-tonics in the same pub but had never used their facilities until then. It was a further 10 days before I was discharged from hospital, still on large doses of corticosteroids and immunosuppressive therapy. I had had no rejection episodes. The most worrying problem was that the donor of my kidney was found to have a small adenocarcinoma of the bronchus on post mortem examination. The consultant in charge of the unit came along a few days after the operation to tell me about this unexpected finding, and said that while he thought that the risk of there being a secondary deposit in the transplanted kidney was very small, the decision was up to me. He said, 'You're in the life and death business, you're used to making decisions and taking the risks'. I decided to keep the kidney, though an article in the *British Medical Journal* one week later about the transplantation of a kidney containing malignant disease which caused the death of the recipient[2] almost made me go back on the decision.

The other problems were routine compared with that. I accepted the dyspepsia from the high steroid dosage, though I was disturbed by the muscle wasting and weakness also due to steroid therapy. I also put up with the nocturia which was accentuated by a minute bladder capacity — after being virtually anuric for 7 years it takes time for bladder capacity to return to full size, and I recall marking out with joy when I could retain

150 ml, later 200 ml and so on. I never have to get up at night to pass urine now.

Another problem during the post-operative period was the possibility of rejection. I was warned to watch out for an increase in the size of the kidney, or tenderness, or an unexpected rise in my temperature. After 11 days I drew my transplant surgeon's attention to an increase in the size of the kidney. He examined it and laughed, commenting that this was the expected physiological hypertrophy. It is very consoling when you know that your transplant has started to grow. However, the increase in size as I became more mobile was difficult to put up with – having a strange object down in my right iliac fossa made walking difficult and totally altered my gait, so much so that my right hip began to ache. I know that the complication of avascular necrosis of the femoral head is more common on the same side as the transplant, and that this has been ascribed to alteration in vascular supply, but I wonder if the stress of walking in a different way is a more important factor.

After discharge from hospital I was taking a pleasant holiday when I began to feel very tired and exhausted, but I did not relate it to the kidney, as there were no other symptoms at the time. After attending for a routine check, I was called back because my plasma creatinine level had risen considerably. I was readmitted – 5 weeks after the operation – and treated for a rejection episode with bolus therapy of high dose methylprednisolone and also radiotherapy to the kidney which was considerably enlarged, firm and slightly tender.

As the episode subsided I suddenly began to spike a high temperature each evening. After 3 days I was certain that I had a viral infection and announced the fact, but was disbelieved. I was subjected to a large series of investigations including sigmoidoscopy and even re-exploration of the kidney after ultrasound had shown a small space behind the kidney which could have contained pus, but in fact did not. My liver was found to be just palpable, but I denied that it was tender since I knew that this would lead to a liver biopsy. The pyrexia continued for several weeks and only subsided on reduction of my immunosuppressie therapy. All the acute investigations were negative although immune complexes were found in the blood, and retrospective investigations of sera which had been collected showed rising titres of Ebstein-Barr virus dating back to the time of the operation, which was presumably due to blood transfusion or to a recrudescence of latent infection, though there was a third, much more remote possibility which I almost completely discarded.

By a strange coincidence, Dr Carmody – the Chairman of this session of the symposium – was in charge of the patient who received the partner kidney from the same donor. I was fascinated to hear that his patient also had a pyrexial illness after transplantation, for which no cause was found. It is interesting to speculate that the infection may have come from the donor; we intend to look further into the story. He also told me last night of the concern that they had about the possibility of malignancy in their recipient; the medical team decided against removal of the kidney without consulting their patient. He still has it, without signs of malignancy.

My main feeling towards the end of my hospital stay was one of relief now that the long period of hesitation and doubt was over. Transplantation itself had resolved the dilemma of whether to have a transplant or not, but it left in its wake a different set of uncertainties which were largely out of my control. By far the main one was the possibility of rejection. The anxiety of the first few weeks gradually receded as the kidney showed signs of taking up permanent residence. Perhaps the strangest feeling of all was the mixed emotion on going back to my treatment room and looking at the machine which, despite any of the moments when I hated it, had been my constant and reliable companion for 7 years.

Later on, when I was back at work, a renal unit technician phoned me asking if they could remove the kidney machine that morning. I told him to go ahead. That evening when I got home, the room looked very bare without the machine and other pieces of equipment. I really felt on my own, rather like someone who has always swum inside his depth, and then goes into deep water where he cannot feel the bottom any more. I also felt more confident then that there was a new future ahead.

Because of the added complications I was off work for just 3 months. I had been warned that my work record (two days off work in 7 years while on haemodialysis) would be much less reliable after renal transplantation due to morbidity from at least some of the complications which so often occur. However, I have been back at work full-time, without missing a day since then, on quite a small dose of the standard therapy (prednisolone 8 mg and azathioprine 100 mg daily) and no other drugs, with good renal function. My latest endogenous creatinine clearance was 52.7 ml/min. I am normotensive, with a haemoglobin which rose to normal within 2 months of operation.

The only continuing complication is of recurrent renal stones, which is a rather unusual problem post-transplantation and possibly under-recognized since symptoms are minimal. There is no sensation of renal colic, because the transplanted kidney and ureter have no nerve supply.

The future now looks good, though I am still concerned about the long-term complications of permanent drug therapy. As a small preventative measure, I have started playing squash regularly in order to minimize the chances of developing osteoporosis. At this distance – just over a year – I am glad to have had my renal transplant. I do not need to tell you that the quality of life is incomparably better; more I think than the rather arbitrary figure of 25% which has been quoted[3].

I took a gamble that has paid off. Apart from quality of life I feel that after 1 year a patient with a functioning transplant who is on a low dose of immunosuppressive therapy probably has a comparable prognosis to that if he had remained on dialysis. If I should have the misfortune to return to dialysis, I would again go through the misgivings I have described, but I would view a further renal transplant with less reluctance.

Many people have said to me, referring to life on haemodialysis, 'I could never go through that kind of experience, I just would never be able to put up with it'. My reply to them all is that if they were actually faced with it, they would manage very well, since there are immense reserves in each of us which often lie dormant until a challenge appears. When such a challenge comes it can be accepted and coped with, particularly if one has faith, the support and affection of family and friends, and a strong sense of purpose in life. In fact, like many of life's misfortunes, the experience of living with renal failure can be character-forming, and can even enrich a person's life.

References

1. Eady, R. A. J. (1973). Why I have not had a kidney transplant after nine and one-half years as a haemodialysis patient. *Transpl. Proc.*, 5, 1115
2. Barnes, A. D. and Fox, M. (1976). Transplantation of tumour with a kidney graft. *Br. Med. J.*, 1, 1442
3. Klarman, H. E., Francis, J. O. and Rosenthal, G. D. (1968). Cost effectiveness analysis applied to the treatment of chronic renal disease. *Med. Care*, 6, 48

15

Some problems of staff stress in dialysis-transplantation units
Mary Brown

15.1 INTRODUCTION

This paper will describe some of the stresses encountered by the staff and patients of a renal dialysis and transplant unit.

The stress is mainly brought about by the type of illness treated, the techniques involved and the isolation of the renal unit from the rest of the hospital.

Staff roles come under conflict if the problems are not brought to frequent and constructive discussion.

Stress itself results in agitation, frustration, sensitivity and resentment. The emotions involved are provoked by occurrences in everyday life. Stress is a part of every working person's life and is certainly not alien to hospitals and renal transplant units. There are, however, some aspects of stress which are more apparent in this speciality than in others.

15.2 SPECIAL PROBLEMS OF PATIENTS

All patients admitted to haemodialysis/transplant units come to be treated for an incurable disease. They are aware that their condition can be treated by haemodialysis, peritoneal dialysis or transplantation along with the necessary adherance to fluid and dietary restrictions, drugs and changes in social and employment habits. Although these patients know that treatment is possible, they are aware that they cannot be cured. Having been informed of their condition, they regard dialysis or transplantation as their last hope. Both patients and relatives are under a great deal of stress, which puts an added strain on their nursing management[1].

The patient who is to be treated by haemodialysis must learn all the technical skills necessary for this procedure, as well as becoming familiar with the required diet, drugs and fluid. He must learn this from the staff of the renal unit, with whom he is going to be closely associated for some years.

The patient who is being treated by transplantation has to undergo surgery and be educated in the use of immunosuppressive drugs and steroid treatment. He has the constant fear of rejection, which may cause him to be agitated and unsure of himself. This has a profound effect on the patient's family. If the transplant is successful, he will not have such close links with the staff of the unit as the dialysis patient does. He must, however, discipline himself to regular checkups at the clinic.

Both dialysis and transplant patients are under a great deal of stress, particularly at the commencement of their treatment. The staff of the renal unit must be educated to appreciate and alleviate the adjustment problems which the patients face.

The main difference between the renal dialysis and transplant unit and other units of the hospital is that here the patient is not just treated with understanding and help in all possible ways, but is also actively involved as a part of the team. He must be included in the decisions concerning his future. Other members to be included in the team are the patient's family, who will be closely concerned in the actual treatment.

15.3   SPECIAL PROBLEMS OF STAFF

Bearing in mind that the patient is automatically included, let us turn to the other members of the team, i.e. the staff of the dialysis/transplant unit.

15.3.1   Team work

The patient comes into contact with the staff from the time that a diagnosis is made. The physician in charge of the patient's diminishing renal function must keep the patient informed of all the possibilities of treatment and truthfully discuss the advantages and disadvantages of each. At the same time he must assess the type of treatment most suitable. The nursing staff may meet the patient while he is in consultation with his physician and have the opportunity to offer an opinion on which course of treatment would best suit him. During this preliminary assessment, all members of the team who are invited to discuss the case are under stress, as the responsibility of a wrong decision regarding treatment at this stage could do irreversible damage to the patient's physical and psychological state. Close contact must be kept with the patient's social worker, who shares the responsibility of helping with the choice of treatment and rehabilitation.

Once the type of treatment has been decided upon, the success of its maintenance depends on the team, including the patient and his family. 'Several disciplines working together do not make a team. Effective team-work requires attention to the process of working together as well as the technical skills each practitioner brings'[2].

As the patient's treatment necessitates a long-term connection with the unit, any inter-staff stress will soon become apparent to him and will affect his relationship with the team.

15.3.2   Nursing staff

The dialysis/transplant unit is staffed by qualified nurses who have a keen interest in the work they do and who have a genuine concern for all the problems the patient comes up against.

Qualified nurses working together have problems amongst themselves, quite apart from the personality clashes which occur in any field of work. Resentment towards each other regarding degrees of responsibility may occur and must be curtailed quickly by group discussion which must be truthful but not hurtful. This problem must be dealt with by the nurse in charge and as many of the team as can be helpful towards establishing priorities for the smooth running of the unit. All helpful opinions must be discussed and, if possible, a satisfactory conclusion reached so tasks are shared in a way that will benefit the whole team.

The nurse in charge of the unit nursing team has many problems. She must diagnose staff stress before it becomes disruptive. Hopefully she can rely on her staff to discuss their problems with her. To enable her to do this, she needs a mature and calm outlook even when the unit is very busy and other matters are awaiting her attention. Even in particularly busy circumstances, she must be available to deal with staff problems, or the result could be detrimental to the care of the patient. The nurse in charge must have the ability to delegate tasks fairly and in return the nurses must be grateful to learn from her example. The nurses working on a dialysis/transplant unit must remember that all final decisions lie with the nurse in charge. As they are familiar with the work of the unit, some with several years' experience, they must help by making suggestions towards any form of treatment or administration known, to their superior. Once the pros and cons of such a suggestion have been considered and a decision made, they must abide by it without bearing any resentment towards another member of staff if they disagree with the final outcome.

The nurse in charge may have help from her Nursing Administrator. In many cases, on the other hand, the Nursing Administrator is inexperienced in this specialization and cannot have a full understanding of the problems involved. This leaves the nurses without senior nursing support. This is not an unfamiliar problem on any specialized unit but it is an added stress.

Team problems do not occur only among nursing personnel. There may well be a disagreement between physician and surgeon or between dietitian and nurse. Again, open discussion can lead to a positive and constructive result and the patient's treatment will continue to be of benefit, hopefully without his realizing there was a conflict. A patient should be included in discussion where two parties have helpful suggestions to make, e.g. regarding diet. For obvious reasons he must be excluded if there is a lack of discipline in the differing personnel.

15.3.3   Medical staff

Team disagreement may be related to a communication gap between the medical staff and the nurses. In all matters of treatment nurses who have high standards and expectations but who do not receive the support of their medical staff will become discontented. In this situation, one of two results may ensue:

(1) The nurses work hard and try to maintain their high standards of care but essentially become frustrated by the lack of involvement of the medical staff. They try not to let their stress affect the patient, but if the situation continues, inevitable breakdown of the team will occur.

(2) They give up the fight. They do not expect too much of their patients. Discipline becomes minimal and the high standard of care will drop. This leads to disillusionment as the nurses know they could do better.

Medical and surgical staff can contribute greatly to the team's success by including all members of nursing staff in decisions regarding treatment. The experienced nurse may have contributory reports to make on a patient's progress which cannot be known to a doctor who visits the patient once or twice a day. The inexperienced nurse will always have something to learn by joining in discussion about her patient. It can be most disheartening to care for a patient for many hours, only to be excluded from any decision about his treatment. Communication between the doctor, the bedside nurse and the patient is most important in this respect.

The experienced dialysis nurse at times has difficulty working with new junior members of the medical team. For the moment, her practical knowledge of dialysis is superior to his. She may have to make a quick decision in an acute case without waiting for his diagnosis. This can cause friction. The consultant in charge will find that this may be solved if new members of the medical staff are educated to respect the experience of the dialysis nurse.

15.3.4   Technical staff

Communications between the technical staff of the unit and the rest of the team must have no barriers. Lack of patient orientation by a technician may result in poor treatment. Alternatively, the rest of the staff must respect the technician's knowledge of his subject and not meddle in this field without consulting him. It is too easy in this situation to end up doing each other's work inefficiently, which is obstructive to the team goal and causes unnecessary friction. 'An important part of nursing on the renal unit is to relieve tension for patients used to living under constant strain'[1].

The staff try to create a relaxed environment for the sake of the patient. An informal atmosphere is encouraged, although difficulty may be encountered trying to maintain mutual respect. New staff and patients may try to take advantage of this informal situation and take some time to adjust to it. This informality may be regarded as unusual by the nursing administration of the hospital and the unit staff may come under criticism. It is difficult to convince the nursing administration that basic nursing standards are maintained even though the nurses are on first name terms with each other and with the patients. Hopefully, it will be realized that the staff are trying to construct a relaxed though respectful relationship with each other and their patients.

15.3.5 Close staff–patient relationships

The staff of the unit come to know the patients and their relatives closely. This is good and the patients trust them with all their problems – medical, social and emotional. In this relationship, the team motive must not be disregarded. A patient and member of staff trying to iron out a problem on a one-to-one basis may be unable to solve it. The member of staff will feel she has failed her patient and the patient still has his problem. Thus two people are under added strain that could be alleviated if the problem had been shared with the team. 'Information must be freely shared. The concept of confidentiality must be altered to include the team, or it will not serve to protect the patient, but to constrict effective teamwork'[3].

Because the staff and patients know each other throughout a period of time they do become friendly, sometimes on a social basis. Staff would not be human if they were not involved with their patients. The death of a patient is upsetting, particularly if the patient has been treated by the unit for some time and is regarded as a friend. The only solution is to be of as much help as possible to the bereaved relatives and try to give some comfort to the other patients on the unit who have been friendly with the deceased. Trying to boost the morale of the other patients and give them renewed confidence in themselves and their treatments brings the team back together again.

A similar stress for patients and staff arises after transplantation. A patient may be discharged from hospital full of health and hope for the future, only to be readmitted in acute rejection. It can be very difficult to hide the staff's disappointment from the patient.

15.3.6 Hepatitis

Dialysis units have the added stress of a possible outbreak of hepatitis at any time. Those who have worked in the speciality for some time will be acutely aware of the possible outcome. The responsibility of controlling the tests for Hepatitis B Antigen on staff, patients and visitors is most important.

15.3.7 Isolation

Visitors to the unit must be restricted, so it functions as an isolated part of the hospital. This is not always good for the morale of the staff. Although they enjoy specializing, there is a danger of forgetting that other parts of the hospital exist, to the extent that new members of staff may only mix socially with those of their own team. This social isolation is not to be encouraged.

15.4 TEACHING AND TRAINING

In the general running of the unit, the staff must become teachers in three areas:

(1) The home-dialysis training scheme.
(2) The training of members of staff.
(3) The education of lay-people with an interest in this field.

Education is an area in which many members of staff are not trained and some find it very difficult.

The training of patients for home-dialysis is rewarding for the most part. However, some patients do not learn quickly and need a great deal of time, patience and understanding. Sometimes a patient does not reach the expected standard despite intensive teaching. The staff do not forget him when he is placed in the home. He is a constant worry, needing many domiciliary visits and many re-calls to clinic for checkups.

Other patients admitted for home-training come to be regarded as unsatisfactory and they must remain on hospital dialysis. The staff, who have tried to train the patient to the best of their ability, feel they have failed and the patient feels disappointed. The staff–patient relationship has to be reassessed before satisfactory hospital dialysis can commence.

15.5 SUMMARY

In summary, though stress does exist in dialysis/transplant units, it is at times more apparent than others. The staff and patients, by striving to be active members of the team, can overcome the problems which arise.

References

1. Richards, G. M. (1974). The emotional aspects of nursing in a renal transplant unit. *Proc. Europ. Dial. Transpl. Nurses Ass.*, 2, 47
2. Kress, H. and Nason, F. (1976). A perspective: the interdisciplinary approach to patients with chronic disease (teaming). *J. Am. Ass. Nephrol. Nurses and Tech.*, 3, no. 1
3. Hayot, M., Kaplan-Nour, A. and Czaczkes, J. W. (1975). Inter-team relationship in a renal unit. *Proc. Europ. Dial. Transpl. Nurses Ass.*, 2, 52

DISCUSSION

B. H. B. Robinson (Birmingham): Dr Henry made an important point about having a purpose in life. In the current unemployment situation with social security provision such that many of the patients who have less well-paid jobs are better off not working than working, there are real problems. However, the effect on morale for patients who are not at work can be quite disastrous and we should perhaps encourage our patients to find something to do.

Carmody: It is important that they do not just stay at home all day.

Robinson: It is obvious that we have not done enough work on what influences patients' lifestyles. I do not know enough about what they can and cannot do.

Henry: It is very difficult to define. It has to be assessed in each individual case. Some will have a virtual 100% rehabilitation and others, for whatever reason, may never get around to being able to work.

F. M. Parsons (Leeds): The EDTA Registry would suggest that evening/ night dialysis gives a better chance for rehabilitation. Perhaps this is one of the advantages of home dialysis versus hospital dialysis. In providing hospital dialysis are we offering our facilities at the right time of day?

Baillie: I looked on time away from work as something temporary, and it was being able to work that really led me to accept the situation. Dr Henry told me that he was able to dialyse through the night, and that he was even able to go to sleep. I could never do that, and I do not think that there are many patients who could plug in and go off to sleep. I found that any movement on the arm would cause blood flow problems.

Henry: I would not have been able to carry out my job if I had not been dialysing at night. At the beginning, when I had an old-fashioned dialyser, we were recommended to dialyse 10 hours, and that takes 12 hours out of the day so I had to sleep on dialysis if I was to work for even 5 days a week.

Parsons: Should day dialysis at hospitals perhaps be shut down?

Henry: It might have an important place for the housewife with a family who wants to be at home in the evening, but for someone who wants to work every day it is better to dialyse late in the evening or overnight.

Baillie: Where one can dialyse late in the evening there is not much of a problem. It does not affect the working day too much.

Parsons: So we are providing a pretty lousy dialysis service in the hospitals?

Henry: There is so much more to be said for home dialysis in terms of independence and mobility in the sense that one can choose when to dialyse, and which nights one wants to dialyse.

A. C. Kennedy (Glasgow): The duration of dialysis is a further pertinent factor. When our unit reduced from two 10-hour spells a week for each patient to three 5-hour spells the number of patients at work increased substantially.

C. Burdett (Leicester): There is evidence that patients on home dialysis seem to return to work more effectively. Perhaps because they have learnt to control their own situations and their own dialysis problems there is greater personal control over everything in life.

Mrs Deirdre E. Jones (London): Is there any way to help relieve the stresses of patients that is not being carried out at the moment?

Mrs M. Brown: Some patients, although we do get them on to home dialysis, do need extra help. They need several domiciliary visits, and this highlights one possible need for 'in-centre' dialysis. A lot of general practitioner medical centres seem to have been built, with clinics for babies and clinics for all kinds of things, and I can see no reason why such centres should not include three or four dialysis rooms where patients could go in and dialyse, and there would be a nurse in the building, and a doctor on the premises in the event of a cardiac arrest. That is all that is needed, and all

the support that the patients want. They want to know that there is somebody medical nearer than a hundred miles who knows vaguely what they
are doing. This would bring in the community services. I do not know what
others in the profession think about bringing the community services into
dialysis.

Ms Jennifer Wedderburn (Nottingham): What about rotating staff from
the renal unit out into the field? The renal unit tends to be rather isolated,
and one tends to forget that there is another part of the hospital. I sometimes wonder whether rotating the staff out of the unit for a period of 6
months might help in some way. In other countries, e.g. America, staff do
move out.

Brown: It probably would help. However, with the work situation being
what it is and the staff situation being what it is, the unit cannot afford to
lose staff for six months of the year.

Wedderburn: And there would be a problem of retraining experienced
staff for the renal unit. However, it is a shame that it cannot be considered.

A. W. Siemsen (Honolulu): Here again the self-care unit is very important.
Our own self-care units run two shifts a day and they will soon be open all
24 hours and patients can come and dialyse at any time that they want.

That also answers the question just asked. Our staff do rotate from
limited care to self-care to acute care. There is a variety of patients and it
does give some relief.

SECTION FIVE

Practical Management
Chairman:
A. C. Kennedy

16

Evaluation of four disposable dialysers
Kathleen Nicholson

16.1 INTRODUCTION

In 1965 the number of regular dialysis patients notified to the EDTA for the whole of Europe was 160. By 1971 this number had risen to 7000 and by 1975 it exceeded 22 000. This dramatic rise has led to logistic and financial problems which have been tackled with varying degrees of success in the different European countries.

By 1975 the budget for regular dialysis in the United Kingdom had risen to £12 million per annum and by now will be much higher. The current period of financial restrictions imposed on the National Health Service has aggravated the situation.

In this setting the introduction of financial savings, even of limited degree, would be helpful. Such savings, however, should not interfere with the efficiency of dialysis to the individual patient as the quality of life in many cases is already sub-optimal.

In the early days of regular dialysis the Kiil dialyser was widely used but was recognized to have several disadvantages. It required space for building and storage and employment of extra personnel. Its use also heightened the risk of cross infection.

In recent years there has been a move towards the use of disposable dialysers, mainly for greater convenience and to lessen the risk of spread of hepatitis. This move has, of course, imposed a greater cost burden with which many Health Authorities have difficulty in coping.

The purpose of this paper is to briefly review the use of three disposable hollow fibre dialysers and one of the disposable Kiil type. Five aspects were examined, namely ease of use, urea and creatinine clearance, ultrafiltration and the cost and efficiency of re-use. Details of the four dialysers are shown in Table 16.1. The Travenol, Nephros (Organon) and Cordis Dow are all hollow fibre kidneys while the Gambro is a disposable Kiil type.

TABLE 16.1   Details of the four dialysers

Manufacturer	Model	Surface area (m^2)	Cost (per dialyser)
Cordis Dow	Mark 4	1.3	£17
Travenol HF	SM1786	1.5	£18
Organon	Nephros 16F.160	1.6	£23
Gambro	Lundia Optima 17 micron	1.0	£15

The Cordis Dow is the only one sterilized by formalin and this has the disadvantage of requiring more complete flushing out by saline prior to use. The burst rate was zero in all cases. This represents a considerable advantage over some earlier dialysers. The volume of saline required to

TABLE 16.2   Washback volume and residual blood volume*

	Cordis Dow	Travenol HF	Nephros	Gambro
Washback volume (ml)	210	300	450	320
Residual blood volume (ml)	2.5	2.5	3.7	3.3

* The figures for washback volume are the mean of six measurements in each case. The values for residual blood volume are those measured by the Newcastle Renal Unit using haemoglobinometry.

virtually clear the dialyser and venous line at end of dialysis is shown in Table 16.2. The Cordis Dow comes out of this comparison best and the Nephros worst with the Travenol and Gambro in an intermediate position. Also shown in Table 16.2 is the residual blood volume which is acceptably low in all cases.

The clearance of urea and creatinine was measured using the standard formula:

$$C = \frac{Q_b(C_a - C_v)}{C_a}$$

C = clearance
Q_b = blood flow (ml per min)
C_a = arterial blood concentration
C_v = venous blood concentration

Figure 16.1 shows the urea clearance of the four kidneys. The Travenol and Gambro are more efficient than the Nephros and Cordis. The creatinine clearance (Figure 16.2) similarly shows the Tavenol and Gambro to

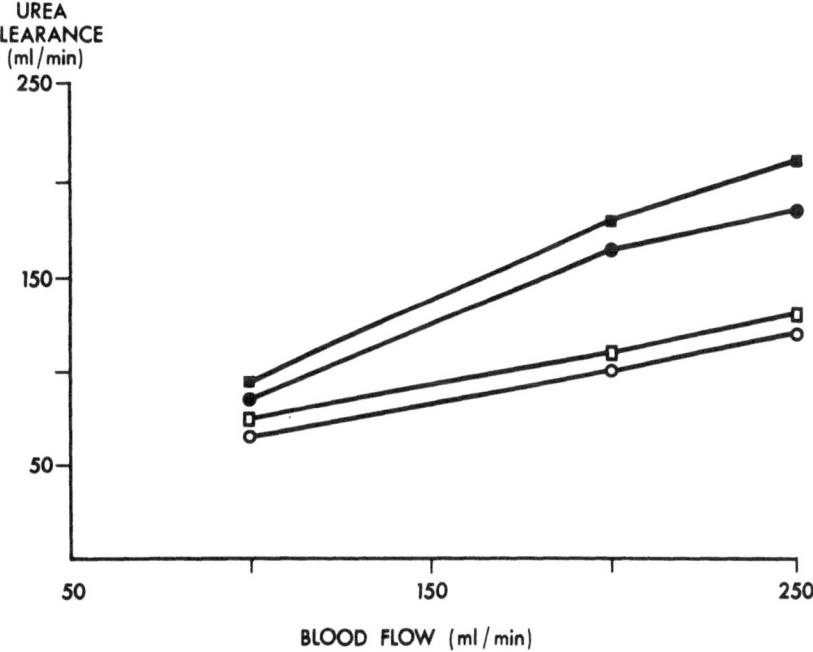

Figure 16.1   Urea clearance at blood flow rates of 100, 200 and 250 ml/min of the Travenol (■), Gambro (●), Nephros (○) and Cordis Dow (□) dialysers. Each value is the mean of six experiments.

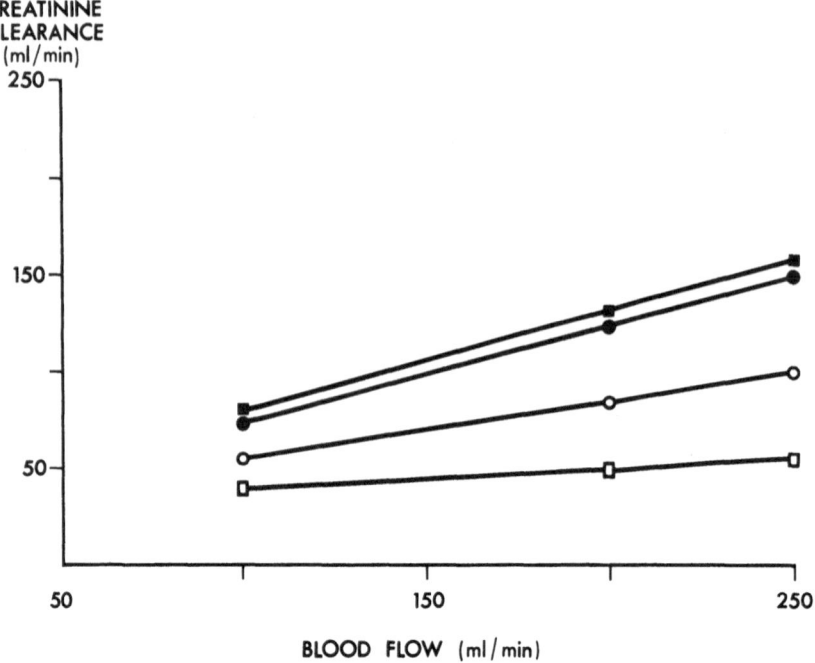

Figure 16.2   Creatinine clearance at blood flow rates of 100, 200 and 250 ml/min of the Travenol (■), Gambro (●), Nephros (○) and Cordis Dow (□) dialysers. Each value is the mean of six experiments

be the best, but in this case the Nephros was superior to the Cordis Dow. Comparison of the ultrafiltration characteristics is shown in Figure 16.3. The highest rate was achieved by the Nephros, with the Travenol next. The rate for the Gambro came next, being much lower than the Travenol at the higher transmembrane pressure, though slightly higher at the lower pressure. These figures relate to the Gambro with 17 micron membrane thickness while it is the 13 micron membrane that is used in most dialysis units. The kidney with the lowest ultrafiltration rate was the Cordis Dow.

16.2   RE-USE OF DIALYSERS

Table 16.3 shows the cost per dialysis related to the number of times the dialyser is re-used. These figures relate only to the dialyser and do not include the lines or other items. Although there is a fairly large variation in cost between the four dialysers, this difference becomes much smaller and therefore less important with re-use.

Also there is little benefit in extending the number of uses beyond six, as

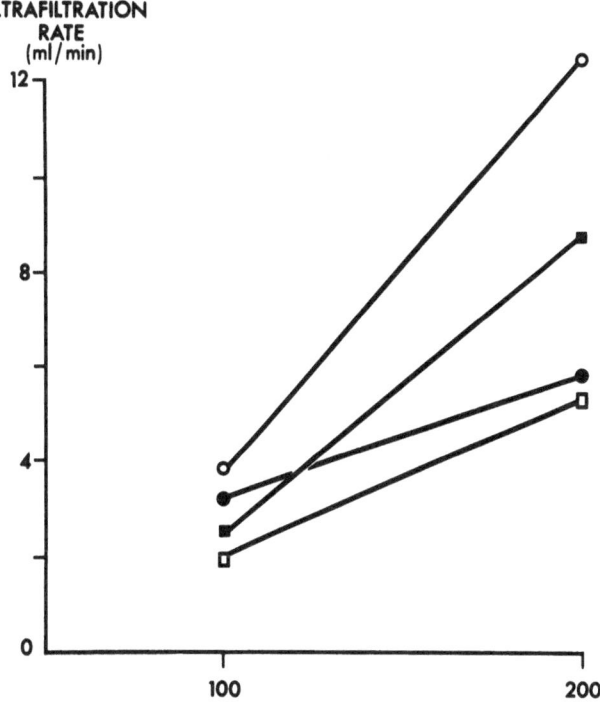

Figure 16.3 Ultrafiltration rate at transmembrane pressures of 100 and 200 mmHg, of the Travenol (■), Gambro (●), Nephros (○) and Cordis Dow (□) dialysers. Each value is the mean of six experiments. The blood flow rate was 100 ml/min

the financial saving per dialysis thereafter becomes small. Taking our unit as an example with 25 patients on thrice weekly dialysis, the annual cost of dialysers when used only once is approximately £71 000. This figure was derived by using the mean of the cost of the four types of dialysers under evaluation. If one used each dialyser six times, the annual cost would

TABLE 16.3 Cost of the dialysers for single, three and six uses

	Single use	Three uses	Six uses
Cordis Dow	£17.00	£5.67	£2.83
Travenol HF	£18.00	£6.00	£3.00
Nephros	£23.00	£7.67	£3.83
Gambro	£15.00	£5.00	£2.50

be less than £12 000, giving rise to a saving each year of £59 000. This saving does not take into account the additional labour costs of re-use but this item is small in relation to the sum saved.

Numerous techniques have been described for re-use. Our method has consisted of flushing out the dialysate compartment with tap water at a pressure of 1000 mmHg (about 20 lb/in^2) and by a form of reverse osmosis this clears the residual blood from the hollow fibres very efficiently. This method cannot be applied to the Gambro and we have not so far re-used this type of dialyser. It should, however, be emphasized that Gambro dialysers are satisfactorily re-used in a number of dialysis units. The use of dialysate to flush out the kidney has been shown to be superior to water and we intend to adopt this method in the future. Following the flushing out, which takes approximately 20 min, the volume of the blood compartment can be measured and this compartment is then filled with 2.5% formaldehyde until the next use (see discussion).

It is important to determine if the efficiency of the dialyser decreases with re-use and our results in relation to this are shown in Table 16.4. One can see that there is no significant decrease in efficiency as measured by urea and creatinine clearances with up to six uses.

TABLE 16.4   Urea and creatinine clearance values during first use and re-use*

	Urea clearance (ml/min)		Creatinine clearance (ml/min)	
	First use	Re-use	First use	Re-use
Travenol HF	210	203 (6)	155	145 (6)
Nephros	124	149 (5)	104	109 (5)
Cordis Dow	128	118 (4)	54	56 (4)

* Each figure is the mean of six experiments. The figures in brackets refer to the number of times each dialyser was re-used. The fact that the Cordis Dow dialyser was used four times in comparison to six times for the Travenol dialyser arose by chance and not design. The blood flow rate for all experiments was 250 ml/min.

16.3   CONCLUSION

Table 16.5 summarizes, using a simple plus system, the relative merits of the four types of dialyser. The Travenol HF and Gambro are best with regard to cost, ease of use and efficiency, but the Travenol HF is much easier to re-use. The Nephros is the least satisfactory in most respects while the Cordis Dow occupies an intermediate position.

To summarize, the currently available hollow fibre dialysers are efficient and easy to use. In addition, their design allows re-use on several occasions without a significant decrease in efficiency. In view of the considerable financial saving, there is a powerful argument for the introduction of re-use in all dialysis units using hollow fibre dialysers.

TABLE 16.5 Summary of the comparative merits of the four types of dialysers

	Ease of use	Cost	Urea clearance	Re-use
Cordis Dow	+ +	+ +	+ +	+
Travenol HF	+ + +	+ +	+ + +	+ + +
Nephros	+ +	+	+ +	+
Gambro	+ + +	+ + +	+ + +	

Key: + Mediocre, + + Satisfactory, + + + Good

DISCUSSION

R. Ahmad (Liverpool): Re-use of the dialyser adds to the time needed for dialysis. The patient who dialyses for 6 hours three times a week will have to put in extra time. What is needed are automatic dialyser washout devices.

A second point. We have had no direction from the DHSS as to where the legal responsibility lies if anything should happen to the patient because the dialyser is re-used. We have been re-using dialysers with considerable success in the case of Travenol and we have also had success in re-using Gambro, and it is all done by automatic re-use devices.

Miss K. Nicholson: We have no automatic re-use machine, although I am aware that they exist.

Ahmad: My patients are re-using dialysers at home, and by using an automatic machine the dialyser can be cleaned and sterilized for re-use in 15 minutes.

Nicholson: The main motive for re-using the kidneys is to save money and that saving can probably be used to employ an additional orderly.

Ahmad: Re-use can even save time.

A. C. Kennedy (Glasgow): Miss Nicholson and Dr Ahmad are really in agreement but the tenor of Dr Ahmad's point should be addressed to a 'Man from the Ministry'. Is there one here?

R. M. Melville (Edinburgh): I am not from the Ministry, but from the Home and Health Department.

Dr Ahmad's point about the responsibility if anything should go wrong because of the re-use of dialysers is a difficult one. I understand from colleagues in the DHSS that having taken bacteriological advice, the general feeling is that the Department cannot recommend the re-use of these disposable dialysers.

Kennedy: If they do not recommend it, can they tolerate it?

Melville: We are not over aware that it is happening.

F. M. Parsons (Leeds): In re-use of dialysers have any pyrexial reactions occurred?

Nicholson: We have not had any.

Parsons: Miss Nicholson said that the dialysers were re-sterilized with $2\frac{1}{2}$% formalin. It should be $2\frac{1}{2}$% formaldehyde. A solution of $2\frac{1}{2}$% formalin is 1% formaldehyde. It is crucial to get the percentages right and there is a difference in terminology between formalin and formaldehyde.

R. J. Winney (Edinburgh): The Cordis Dow is no longer formalin sterilized and is now available in a dry form.
  Secondly, when comparing costs of dialysers, should the variable ultra-filtration rate be taken into account? In some patients this requires replacement with as much as 3 litres of saline, which costs money, and this should be taken into account in comparing the costs of the various dialysers.

Nicholson: I know that Cordis Dow are now dry, but when the paper was prepared we were still using the old Cordis Dow.
  Secondly, while we have been ultrafiltrating our patients, they have not in fact required saline.

J. S. Robson (Edinburgh): Miss Nicholson gave the Travenol three stars for re-use. What characteristic justifies that? Is it ease, or cost, or clearance?

Nicholson: Clearance. We can re-use the Travenol more times than we can re-use the Cordis or the Nephros.

Ahmad: The Travenol is cheaper than the Cordis and has slightly higher clearances for creatinine and urea. I have re-used dialysers as many as 12 times with no trouble, but the point should be made that if a dialyser is re-used more than six times then the amount of money saved is minimal compared to the effort which must be put in it.

Ms Briony Furlong (London): Why has Miss Nicholson not re-used the Gambro? Were there any specific difficulties?

Nicholson: To begin with we did have some difficulty in re-using the Gambro, and we decided to leave it to a later date and to try to re-use it again.

Mrs Deirdre E. Jones (London): Would Miss Nicholson define her methodology of re-use.

Nicholson: Briefly. When the patient comes off dialysis the technicians flush out the dialyser with saline. Residual blood volume is measured, and on that will depend whether it is re-used again. It is then flushed out clear and filled with formaldehyde $2\frac{1}{2}\%$.

Wallace (Glasgow): One of the reported complications of re-using dialysers is that the patients may develop an anti-N, an antibody to the red cell antigens. There have been reports from Australia and from America, and so far it would seem that this complication only occurs where formalin is used for sterilisation. The point was considered in Glasgow before Miss Nicholson started to re-use dialysers.

Does anybody know whether this complication has been observed in Britain?

J. D. Briggs (Glasgow): We ourselves have not re-used enough to measure these antibodies before and after so we have no direct experience. I am not aware of any figures from British units. There seems to have been some debate on this and a Paper was read at EDTA a couple of years back which referred to these antibodies being found after even a single use. I do not know whether it is at all certain how much part re-use plays in the production of these antibodies. There has been some concern about it in relation to possible effects in such patients should they be transplanted. However, we do not know the answer.

I believe that we could get round it. It is a cold antibody, and if one was careful not to transplant a kidney without first warming it up that would probably avoid any risk.

A. W. Siemsen (Honolulu): Our series on measuring antibodies in coil re-use was published in 1976[1] and it clearly demonstrated that the incidence was already high in patients with higher serum creatinines. It was a function of the uraemic process, or something else, but not the re-use. There was no difference between those patients whose dialysers were re-used and those whose dialysers were not re-used. It was already high in people that had creatinines of 10, 11 and 12 but were never dialysed, and there was no difference between patients on peritoneal dialysis and haemo-dialysis. I know of no clinical significance to anti-M.

M. Ward (Newcastle): We have seen anti-M and anti-N antibodies in formalin re-used Meltec multipoint dialysers, which is what we use rou-tinely in our patients. So far we have seen no problems clinically after transplantation.

Ms Jennifer Wedderburn (Nottingham): How many times after re-use is the maximum effective clearance, comparable with the first time used?

Briggs: We have not re-used kidneys excessively. As Dr Ahmad pointed out earlier, the financial saving does not make it worth re-using more than six times. We did re-use a few of the kidneys seven or eight times, but we stopped because it did not seem worth going on. Our figures show no significant fall-off in performance if they are used six times.

There is perhaps some variance with the Newcastle figures.

Ward: We are suprised that people can produce such good clearances after multiple re-use. it may be that their control of heparinization is very much better than we practise in Newcastle. We have had trouble with the Cordis Dow 4's and 5's. They have shown a tremendous drop off in clearance after re-use, even one, two, or three times.

We did re-use the Travenol. To be fair we found that this was the best one to re-use and the clearances were high, but there was still a drop off. We have only re-used them three times. We are financed by the Depart-ment and they are not that interested in trying to save money. We are trying to persevere and we may test some of the automatic re-use equip-ment if we can get our hands on it.

Reference

1. Nolph, K. D., Husted, F. C., Sharp, G. C. and Siemsen, A. W. (1976). Anti-bodies to nuclear antigens in patients undergoing long-term haemodialysis. *Am. J. Med.*, **60**, 673

17

Developments in vascular access
A. McL. Jenkins

17.1 INTRODUCTION

In the last decade there has been considerable progress in techniques of secondary vascular access. The primary methods, which include the Quinton–Scribner Teflon shunt and the Brescia–Cimino arteriovenous fistula at the wrist, are applicable to most patients requiring haemodialysis with intact peripheral vessels. However, many dialysis units have increasing numbers of patients with failed primary access or who have absent peripheral vessels owing to arterial or venous occlusive disease. More patients in this group are being encountered as dialysis units relax their criteria of acceptance regarding age and conditions such as diabetes.

The secondary forms of access include alternative positioning of Teflon shunts and arteriovenous fistulae but recently much attention has been focused on vascular conduits used as subcutaneous grafts. Autologous, homologous and heterologous conduits have been used and lately there has been renewed interest in pure prosthetic materials with some encouraging clinical reports.

Whereas in past years the patient who was coming to the end of his 'shunt life' was an accepted entity, the numerous techniques now available ensure that some form of reasonably safe and reliable vascular access can be instituted.

17.2 FORMULATION OF AN ACCESS POLICY

Whatever form of long-term access is selected the patient's individual needs must be considered. Of basic importance is to place the access at a site convenient for use by the dominant hand. When end-stage renal failure can be anticipated a wrist arteriovenous fistula is the simplest and best form of vascular access. Its timely formation may make a Teflon shunt with its attendant complications unnecessary. However, if dialysis is urgent an ankle Teflon shunt usually proves satisfactory until an arteriovenous fistula becomes usable.

In certain categories of patient one or both of the two primary forms of access may not be possible. These include patients with (*a*) Occluded arteries and veins at ankle and wrist due to previous failed vascular access or obliterative vascular disease. (*b*) Weak pulses at ankle or wrist. Poor flow and occlusion is likely to occur if such vessels are used. (*c*) Heavily calcified vessels. Such vessels may be difficult to suture and rarely develop good flow. They are commonly seen in diabetics. (*d*) Unsuitable anatomical configuration of forearm veins. The veins may lie deeply in subcutaneous tissue or may be multiple. This usually becomes evident on failure of a wrist arteriovenous fistula to mature and is commonest in women.

In these situations some form of secondary access will be required. It is preferable to attempt a simple secondary procedure in the first instance such as a brachial arteriovenous fistula before embarking on the more major operation of insertion of a vascular conduit.

Patients who have functioning conduits should be reviewed at intervals because of the well known tendency for stenosis to develop in association with some types. It is better to diagnose such lesions either clinically or angiographically in time to carry out corrective surgery rather than lose an irreversibly clotted graft.

17.3 COMPLICATIONS OF VASCULAR ACCESS PROCEDURES

Access operations on blood vessels are attended by most of the risks inherent in vascular surgery. In addition there are certain special complications relating to arteriovenous shunting of blood and to the use of dialysis cannulae.

17.3.1 Infection

Infection in association with vascular access operations is potentially of serious significance. If introduced at the time of operation it is difficult to eradicate, especially when vascular prostheses are involved, and secondary haemorrhage may occur from anastomoses. Removal of the prosthesis is likely to be necessary. Local infection at cannulation sites is a moderately common complication. It often responds to conservative treatment but can also result in severe haemorrhage.

17.3.2 Aneurysms

Aneurysmal dilatation of veins adjacent to an arteriovenous fistula is comparatively common but is not often attended by serious complications. Dilatation of saphenous vein grafts occurs especially if the veins were initially varicose.

False aneurysms may result from cannulation of vascular grafts too soon after implantation before the subcutaneous tissues have become adherent to the outer surface of the graft.

17.3.3 Graft stenosis and thrombosis

Occlusion of a graft in the early postoperative period is likely to be due to faulty technique or selection of vessels with poor flow. Occlusion of a well established graft may be caused by stenosis in the graft itself or in the draining vein. Outflow stenosis results in an excessively turgid graft with an exaggerated pulse. Marked bleeding also tends to occur on removal of cannulae from such grafts at the end of dialysis.

17.3.4   High output cardiac failure

Shunts and arteriovenous fistulae inevitably reduce peripheral resistance and in susceptible patients cardiac failure may occur[1]. However, this is comparatively uncommon and we have not so far seen it in our own patients. Limitation of the size and number of fistulae is probably important in prevention.

17.3.5   Limb ischaemia

This is commonest in association with more proximal limb fistulae[2] but also occurs with fistulae at wrist level[3]. Vascular disease in diabetes may exacerbate ischaemia distal to a fistula and has been described by Buselmeier[4]. In diabetics who have concomitant distal vascular disease the radial artery beyond the fistula should therefore be ligated to prevent retrograde flow of arterial blood from the hand to the fistula.

17.3.6   Hand swelling

This occurs comparatively frequently and is due to retrograde arterialization of a vein. It is occasionally marked and in our own series one patient with retrograde arterialization from a wrist arteriovenous fistula developed gross swelling and ulceration of the fingers. Ligation of the affected vein resolved the symptoms.

17.4   VASCULAR ACCESS TECHNIQUES

17.4.1   The Teflon shunt

The technique described by Quinton, Dillard and Scribner[5] in 1960 made long-term haemodialysis possible and was a major advance in treatment of renal failure. The principle is familiar to all dialysis units as are the associated complications leading to shunt failure. The shunt with its external Silastic tubing and Teflon vascular tips is usually inserted into the

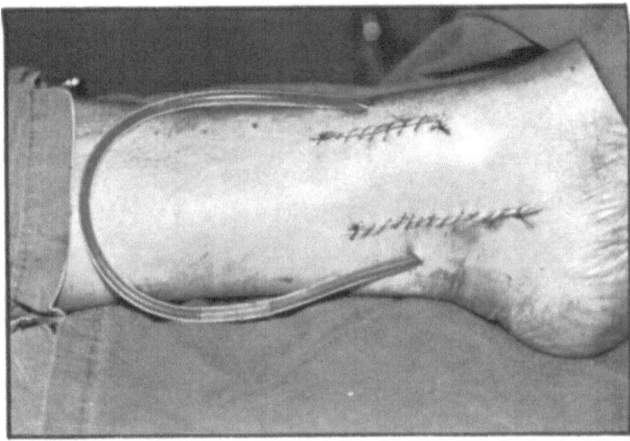

Figure 17.1
Teflon–Silastic
shunt at ankle

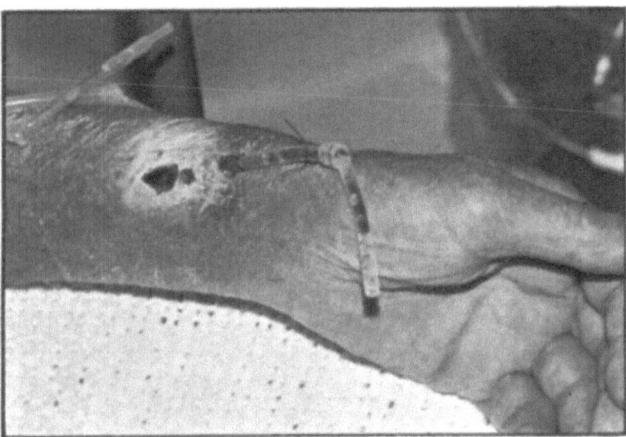

Figure 17.2
Teflon–Silastic shunt with
overlying skin necrosis

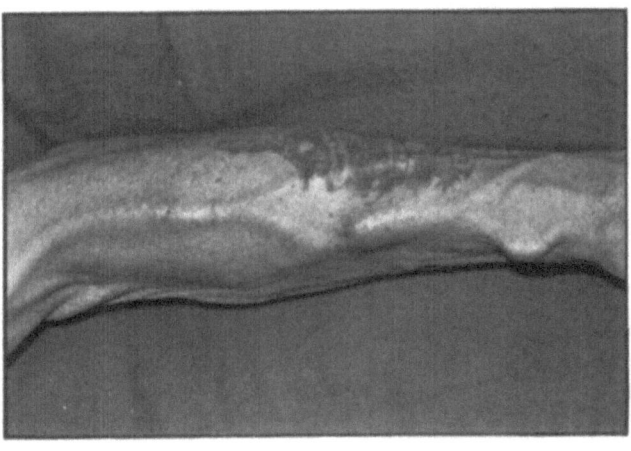

Figure 17.3
Forearm veins in mature
radiocephalic fistula

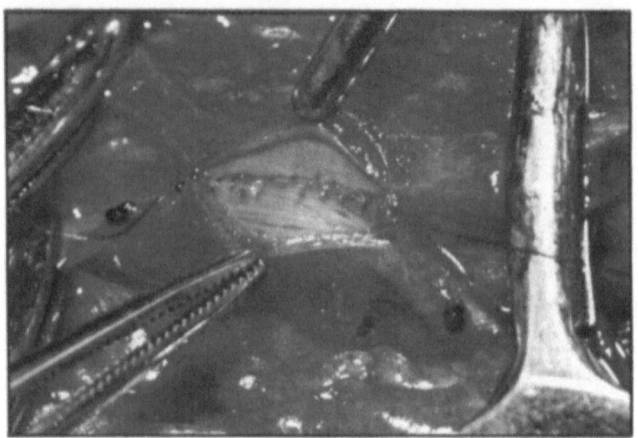

Figure 17.4
Side-to-side anastomosis
between radial artery and
cephalic vein

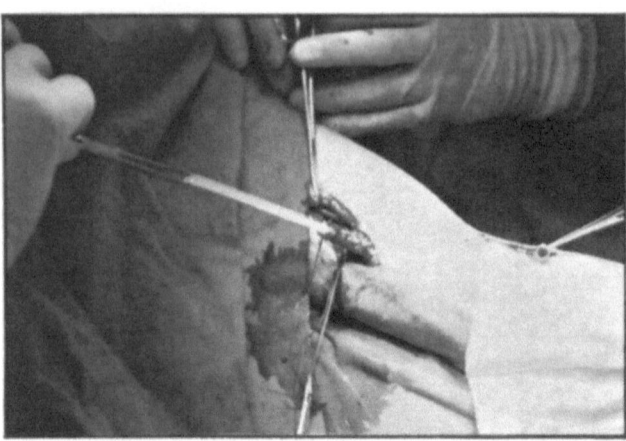

Figure 17.5
Removal of core from
mature Sparks mandril

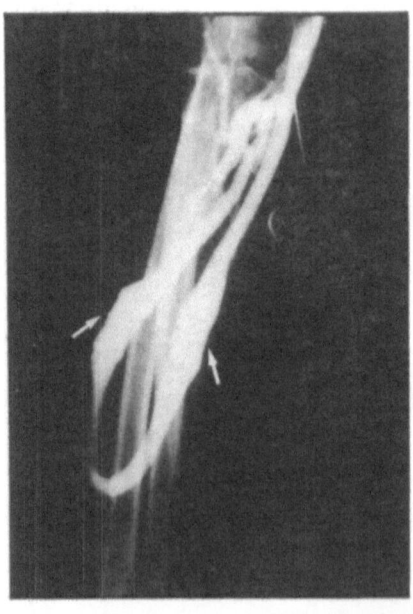

Figure 17.6
Aneurysmal dilatation (arrowed) produced
by conventional dialysis cannulae in a
Sparks mandril

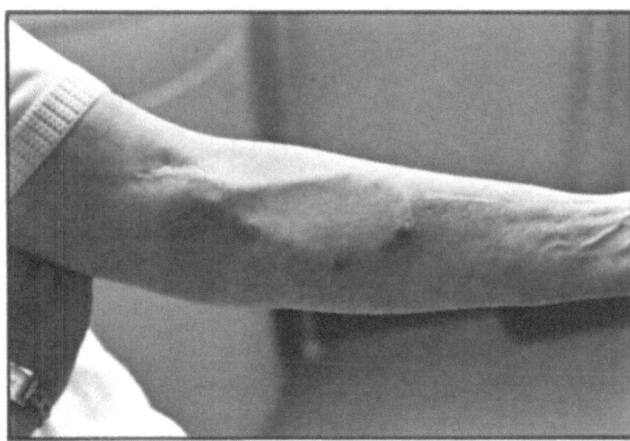

Figure 17.7
Mature forearm saphenous
vein graft loop

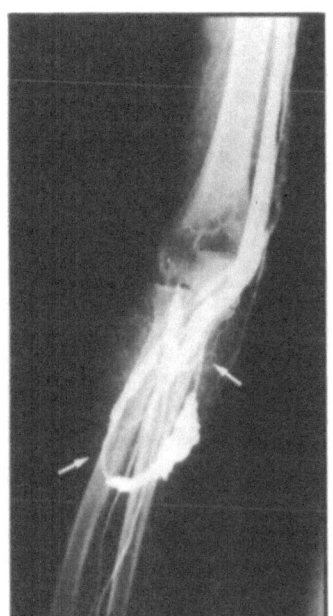

Figure 17.8 Angiogram showing two stenotic
segments (arrowed) produced by
cannulation in a forearm saphenous
vein graft loop

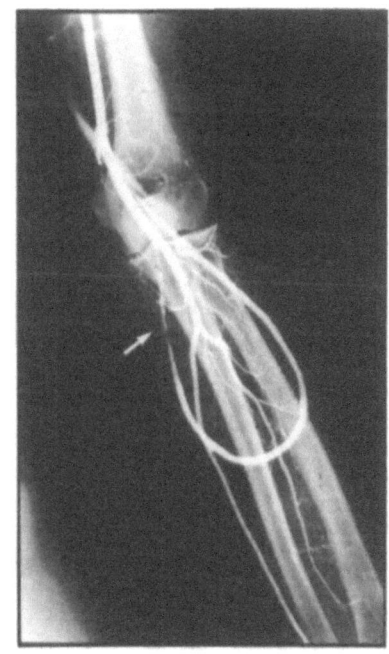

Figure 17.9
Angiogram showing diffuse stenosis
(arrowed) in a forearm saphenous
vein graft loop

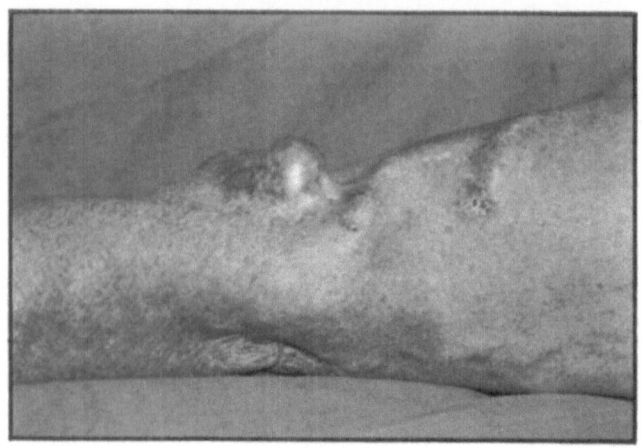

Figure 17.10
Aneurysmal dilatation of
a vein graft

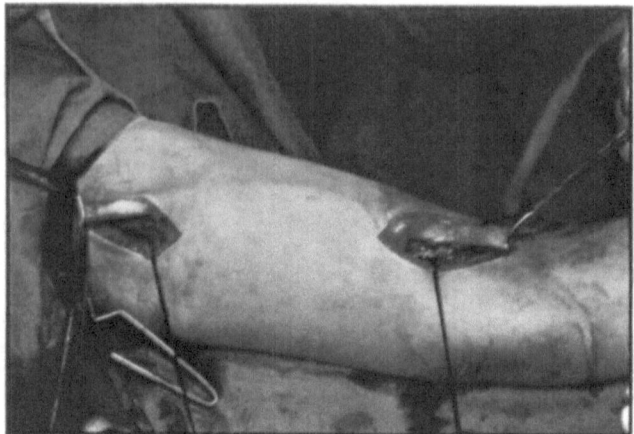

Figure 17.11
Subcutaneous positioning
of an upper arm bovine
heterograft

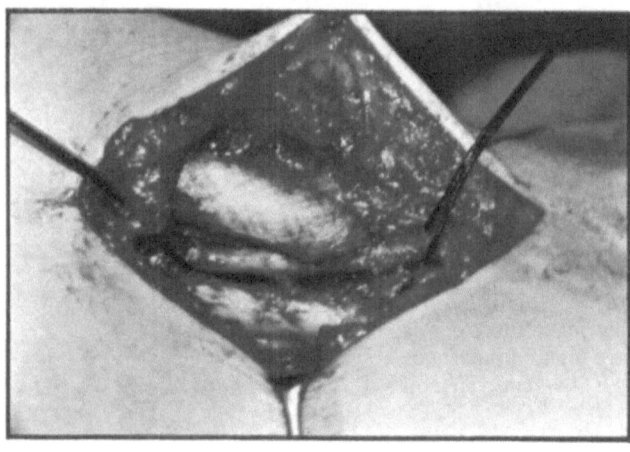

Figure 17.12
Anastomosis of bovine
heterograft to the brachial
artery

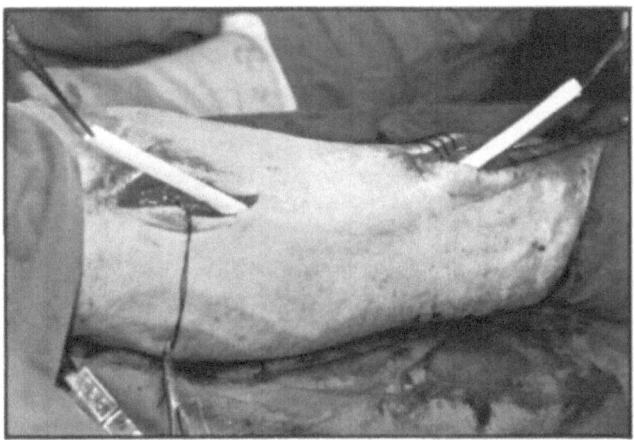

Figure 17.13
Subcutaneous positioning of
a straight forearm expanded
PTFE graft

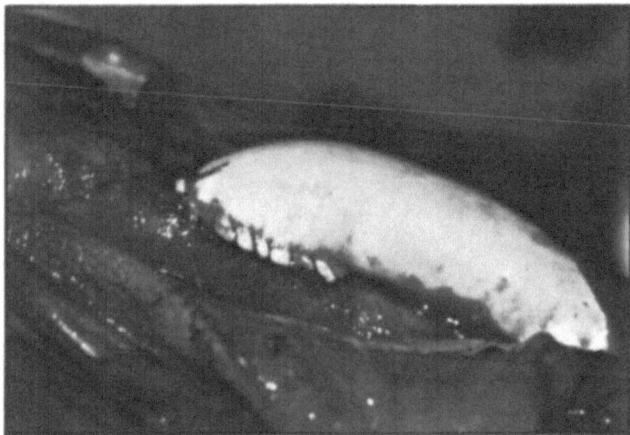

Figure 17.14
Arterial anastomosis of an
expanded PTFE graft

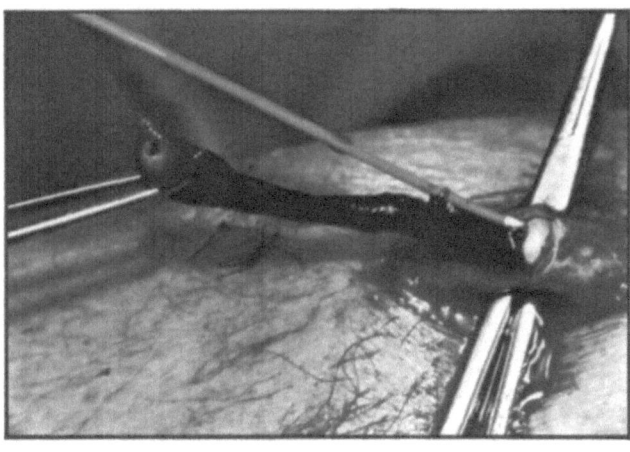

Figure 17.15
Thrombectomy by balloon
catheter of an occluded
expanded PTFE graft

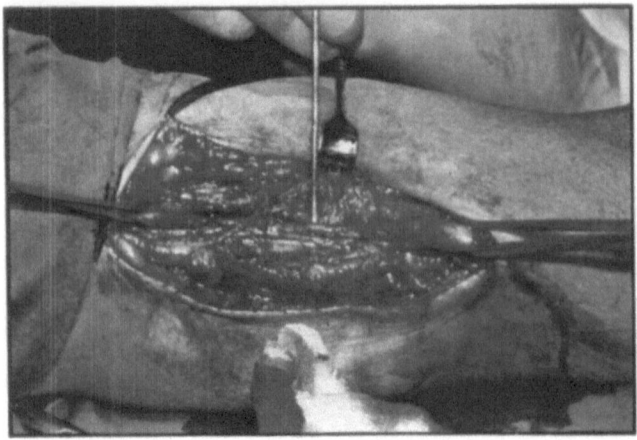

Figure 17.16
Operative appearance of venous stenosis (at pointer between expanded PTFE graft anastomosis (taped right) and normal draining vein (taped on left)

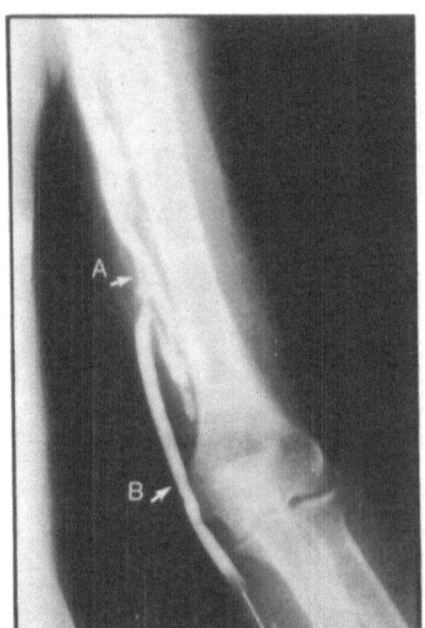

Figure 17.17
Angiogram showing stenosis (A) of run-off vein adjacent to anastomosis of expanded PTFE graft (B)

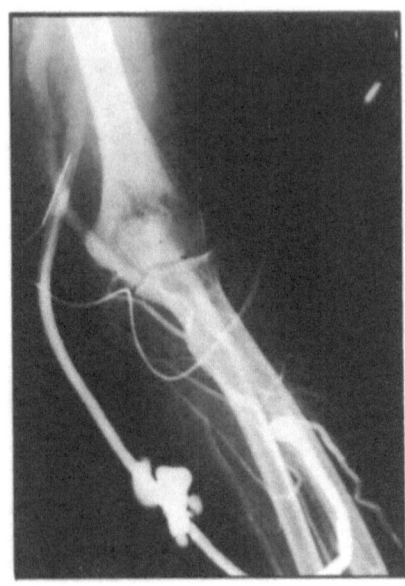

Figure 17.18
Cannulation aneurysm in a PTFE graft

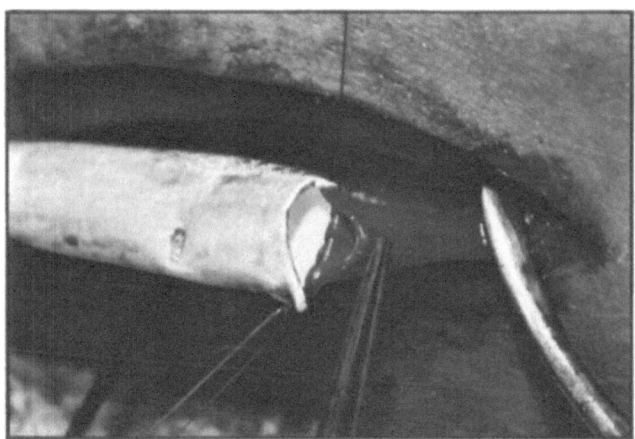

Figure 17.19
End-to-end anastomosis of
expanded PTFE graft

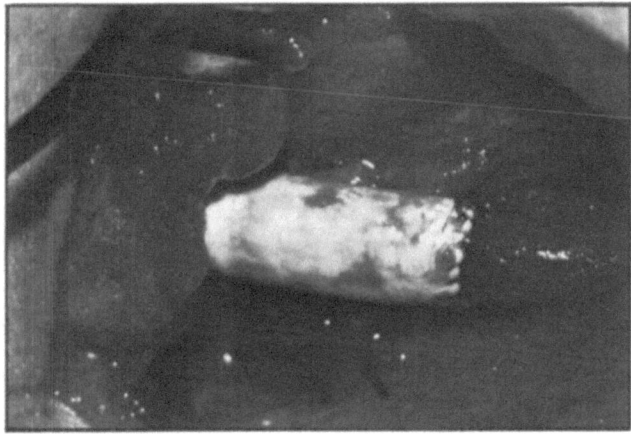

Figure 17.20
Completed anastomosis
between expanded PTFE
graft and axillary vein

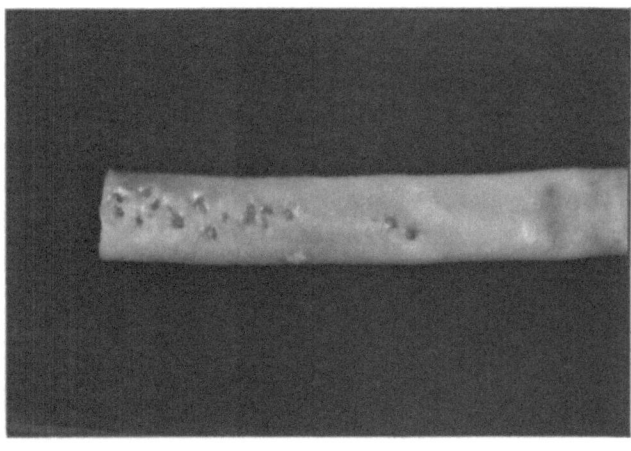

Figure 17.21
Dialysis needle holes in
excised expanded PTFE graft

posterior tibial artery and long saphenous vein at the ankle (Figure 17.1). Numerous other sites are possible but the wrist is avoided if long-term dialysis is likely in order to save the vessels for a radiocephalic arterio-venous fistula. Insertion into the brachial artery gives good flow but spoils distal arteries for future use. Other sites have been described including the inferior epigastric artery and vein[6]. To avoid necessity of arterial ligation around the shunt tip a short segment vein graft can be anastomosed to the side of an artery and used to contain the tip so preserving arterial con-tinuity. This technique has been described with the femoral artery[7], and the brachial artery[8].

Precise surgical technique is essential for good shunt function. Forcing a too large tip into an artery strips up a cuff of intima leading to throm-bosis whereas a 'temperamental' shunt is often caused by vessel tip angu-lation. Unless the Silastic tubing is well buried in subcutaneous tissue skin necrosis may occur while a haematoma round the tubing encourages infection (Figure 17.2).

In spite of good operative technique most of these shunts fail in 3–6 months. The usual causes are stenosis leading to thrombosis in the vein adjacent to the vessel tip and infection, which occurs in a range of 17–50% of patients[9].

17.4.2 Arteriovenous fistulae

The standard side-to-side radiocephalic anastomosis at the wrist was described by Brescia et al.[10], and is the procedure of choice for long-term haemodialysis (Figures 17.3, 17.4). Anastomosis end of vein to side of artery is used by some to prevent distal arterialization of the veins of the hand which on occasion produces severe swelling[11]. Numerous variations of the technique have been described along with alternative sites. One of the most useful when the forearm vessels are unsuitable is the brachio-cephalic fistula[12,13].

17.4.3 Sparks mandril

This device was originally designed for peripheral vascular surgery but has been used subsequently for vascular access[14]. It consists of a solid Silastic rod covered with a double layer of loosely knitted Dacron and provides a method of 'growing' an artificial blood conduit in situ. The mandril is buried subcutaneously in the desired position and becomes incorporated into the tissues, the ends being placed near a previously located artery and vein. Six weeks after implantation the ends are mobilized and the Silastic rod is withdrawn, leaving a smoothly lined conduit (Figure 17.5). The mature mandril is then anastomosed to the vessels and can then be used for haemodialysis cannulation.

The obvious disadvantage of the mandril is the 6-week growing period, which is always inconvenient, and two operations are needed. We have found that it is not always technically simple to anastomose the rather bulky ends to smallish limb vessels. We have used conventional cutting dialysis needles and have noted consistent development of aneurysms of the conduits in the areas penetrated (Figure 17.6). Anastomotic aneurysms have also developed in those longstanding mandrils which have had to be re-anastomosed to bypass dilations caused by needling.

Others have found the patency rate among mandrils to be inferior to autogenous vein grafts[15] and this means of access is now used less frequently.

17.4.4   Vein grafts

Since the original description of a forearm loop constructed from the long saphenous vein[16] numerous other forms of the graft have been used. Autogenous grafts are most commonly employed but others have shown that preserved homografts also function[17, 18].

The suitability of various veins has been described by Bell and Calman[19]. The long saphenous vein in the thigh is consistently the best for use as a graft though occasionally the distended diameter is poor and if less than 5 mm we employ other means of access. The cephalic vein in the upper arm is also a good graft source but the obvious scarring and discomfort which follow its removal discourage its frequent use. The external jugular veins are also a possible source of graft material.

17.4.4.1   *Graft configurations*

(a) *Forearm grafts* – The most commonly employed forearm grafts are loops arising from the brachial artery near the elbow with return to an adjacent vein (Figure 17.7). They usually function well, but straight forms between the brachial artery and a distal vein are also satisfactory[20]. In our experience the loop types have better patency. Artery to artery grafts have been described between the brachial and radial artery[11].

(b) *Upper arm grafts* – Upper arm grafts are less convenient from the patient's point of view but this form between the brachial artery distally and basilic vein proximally (or vice versa) develop very high flow rates. Such grafts should arch anteriorly to overlie the biceps. Proximity to the neurovascular bundle may result in nerve damage from faulty cannulation and in our experience with various conduits in this position severe local discomfort can occur during dialysis presumably from pressure of the needles on the nerve trunks.

(c) *Lower limb grafts* – Self cannulation of lower limb grafts is easy as both of the patient's hands are free. Transection of the saphenous vein distally in the thigh with anastomosis of the proximal cut end to the femoral artery near the groin results in a high flow loop[21]. It has the technical advantage that an arterial anastomosis only is required.

17.4.4.2   Complications of vein grafts

(a) *Thrombosis* – The incidence of thrombosis of vein grafts is probably lower than with other types of conduit. In our own recent series of 27 vein grafts, of which most were forearm types, there were four occlusions and on each occasion the graft was lost (Table 17.1). We now carry out intermittent check angiograms to identify correctable lesions which might cause

TABLE 17.1   27 Autogenous saphenous vein grafts for vascular access. Thrombotic loss (follow-up 2 months to 2 years)

Graft form	No. inserted	No. occlusions	No. lost (weeks)
Forearm straight	5	1	1 (12)
Forearm loop	19	3	3 (20; 36; 57)
Upper arm straight	2	0	0
Thigh loop	1	0	0
Totals	27	4	4

thrombosis and have demonstrated two types of stenosis. One occurs adjacent to the needling sites giving two localized stenotic segments in a graft (Figure 17.8). The other is a diffuse stenosis with no clear termination point situated in a part of the graft not used for needle insertion (Figure 17.9). The former in some degree was present in the majority of the longstanding grafts, but the diffuse type was seen in two of the 27.

In our experience thrombosis may also develop when a faulty technique is used for removing needles. If excess digital pressure is used to stop bleeding graft flow ceases entirely and clotting results if this is maintained. This applies to all vascular access grafts but does not seem to ocur with arteriovenous fistulae possibly because communicating veins maintain some flow. Patients whose access has been changed from a fistula to a conduit should be appropriately warned.

(b) *Aneurysmal dilation* – Aneurysmal dilation has occurred in some grafts in our own series but has produced surprisingly little disturbance to graft function (Figure 17.10). There seems little danger of severe haemorrhage from the dilated areas and unsightliness may be the main indication for repair or alteration in the means of access.

(c) *Haemorrhage* – Severe haemorrhage may result if an infected focus develops at a cannula puncture site. This occurred with one patient in our series who repeatedly cannulated the same spot. Dramatic haemorrhage necessitated ligation of the segment but access function was preserved by means of a local bypass graft.

17.4.5   Bovine artery heterograft

In 1970 Rosenberg[22] described the use of modified bovine carotid arteries in arterial surgery and since then many others have used this graft for vascular access[23-28]. The results were reviewed by Rosenberg[29]. The grafts which are treated with ficin and with glutaraldehyde tanning are not significantly antigenic[30]. When implanted they incite a fibroblastic reaction unlike the cellular inflammatory response of untreated heterografts. They can be obtained in diameters suitable for vascular access, though the smallest easily obtainable diameter (7 mm) is on the large side for distal limb grafting.

Straight forms between an artery and vein or artery and artery[31] appear to give a higher patency rate than loops. Haimov[27] found that three of four loops clotted soon after surgery. Favourable sites are in the thigh and upper arm though forearm straight forms may also be acceptable[23]. We have used these grafts in a small number of patients in the upper arm and have had no complications over a period of $2\frac{1}{2}$ years (Figures 17.11, 17.12). In some centres the bovine graft is considered to be the best means of secondary vascular access provided that loop forms are avoided[24,26,32].

Bovine and Dacron grafts have been shown to be equally susceptible to experimental infection with *Staphylococcus aureus* but anastomotic disruption occurred more frequently with bovine material[33]. Several workers have reported infected foci at needling sites[24,32], and there is a risk of formation of false aneurysms. There is some evidence to suggest that bovine grafts should not be used for three weeks from the time of insertion as the incidence of aneurysms may thereby be increased.

17.4.6   Expanded polytetrafluoroethylene (PTFE) Gore-Tex vascular prostheses

In the last year there have been reports of use of this material for vascular access, some of which give promising results[34-37].

The microstructure of expanded PTFE consists of nodes interconnected by fine fibrils. The open formation allows rapid cellular ingrowth and the grafts become completely incorporated into the tissues. In contrast to bovine grafts the lumen acquires a continuous neointima and this may be a factor contributing to high patency rates when the prostheses are used for reasons other than vascular access[38,39].

We have conducted a pilot study on the use of expanded PTFE (Gore-Tex)* grafts for vascular access (Table 17.2). The aims were: (a) To assess their surgical suitability for anastomosis to the medium and smaller vessels of the limbs. (b) To establish which was the best graft configuration with regard to patency. (c) To assess the effect of dialysis needles on the graft walls.

TABLE 17.2   PTFE Gore-Tex vascular access grafts. Thrombotic loss (follow-up 1 month to $1\frac{1}{2}$ years)

Graft form	No. inserted	No. occlusions	No. lost (weeks)
Forearm straight	2	2	2 (4; 50)
Forearm loop	5	7	1 (17)
Upper arm straight	4	0	0
Thigh loop	2	1	0
Segmental replacement	1	0	0
Totals	14	10	3

Prostheses of 6 mm internal diameter were used in lengths varying between 19 and 58 cm. The period of follow-up was between 1 month and $1\frac{1}{2}$ years. Fourteen grafts were inserted in 13 patients. The majority were in the forearm (Figure 17.13), but latterly we favoured upper arm types. There was one thigh loop from the common femoral artery to the long saphenous vein, and one segmental replacement of a stenotic area in a forearm loop.

The grafts were highly satisfactory from a purely surgical point of view. Fine anastomoses were simple to fashion and there was no tendency for the material to fray (Figure 17.14).

* W. L. Gore and Associates UK Ltd, Pitreavie Industrial Estate, Dunfermline, Fife

Both forearm types had a high incidence of thrombosis with nine occlusive episodes among seven grafts. Thrombectomy by balloon catheter (Figure 17.15) was often successful but three of these grafts were lost. No occlusions occurred earlier than 4 weeks postoperatively. Graft angiograms or direct inspection at operation demonstrated marked stenosis (1–3 cm in length) in the recipient veins of all grafts just central to the end-to-side graft to vein anastomoses (Figures 17.16, 17.17). There were no other complications apart from infection in one occluded graft which was probably introduced by attempted needling, and aneurysm formation in a segment subjected to needling in another (Figure 17.18).

Following this initial experience we placed the venous ends of the grafts into larger proximal limb veins using end-to-end anastomosis to reduce turbulence. The four upper arm straight grafts originated from the brachial artery just proximal to the cubital fossa with venous anastomosis to the transected origin of the axillary vein (Figures 17.19, 17.20). So far all grafts have functioned normally without angiographic evidence of run-off vein stenosis. We now routinely use long-term antiplatelet drugs for these patients and while there is no definite evidence that they are of value in this situation others have demonstrated that they reduce the incidence of thrombosis in Teflon shunts which also develop run-off vein stenosis[40, 41].

Excised grafts were completely infiltrated with fibrous tissue with continuous smooth neointima except at the large defects made by needles which were filled with granulation tissue (Figure 17.21). These defects could be seen on angiography but there were no clinically evident aneurysms. Sections taken through stenotic veins adjacent to graft anastomoses showed platelet deposition and intimal hyperplasia which often reduced the lumen by up to 80%.

Baker et al.[35] reported a series of 84 expanded PTFE grafts (IMPRA)* and among 64 forearm types there were only 15 occlusive episodes. In only one of these was stenosis of the run-off vein cited as a cause of the occlusion. The disparity between these and our own findings is not clear, though the follow-up period in our series is longer. Kaplan et al.[36] reported a smaller series which included 13 forearm grafts (IMPRA) with no occlusions. The period of follow-up however was again shorter than our own.

In spite of our initial problems with expanded PTFE grafts we regard them as potentially the most acceptable alternative to autogenous vein grafts. Their handling properties are superior to those of bovine hetrografts and a more suitable range of diameters is available. When used as straight grafts proximally in the limb the patency may equal that of vein

* International Medical Prosthetic Research Association Inc., 4209 536th Place, Phoenix, Arizona

grafts and their use avoids the inevitable scarring associated with harvesting the saphenous vein.

References

1. Ahearn, D. J. and Maher, J. F. (1972). Heart-failure as a complication of hemodialysis arteriovenous fistula. *Ann. Intern. Med.*, 77, 201
2. Matold, W., Kastagir, B., Stevens, L. E., Chrysanthakopoulos, S., Weaver, D. H. and Klinkmann, H. (1971). Neurovascular complications of brachial arteriovenous fistula. *Am. J. Surg.*, 121, 716
2. Storey, B. G., George, C. R. P., Stewart, J. H., Tiller, D. J., May, J. and Shiel, A. G. R. (1969). Embolic and ischemic complications after anastomosis of radial artery to cephalic vein. *Surgery*, 66, 325
4. Buselmeier, T. J., Najarian, J. S., Simmons, R. L., Rattazzi, L. C., von Hartitzsch, B., Callender, C. O., Goetz, F. C. and Kjellstrand, C. M. (1973). A-V fistulas and the diabetic: Ischemia and gangrene may result in amputation. *Trans. Am. Soc. Artif. Intern. Organs*, 19, 49
5. Quinton, W. E., Dillard, D. and Scribner, B. H. (1960). Cannulation of blood vessels for prolonged hemodialysis. *Trans. Am. Soc. Artif. Intern. Organs*, 6, 104
6. Kauffman, Jr, H. M. (1975). Deep inferior epigastric arteriovenous shunt for hemodialysis. *Surgery*, 78, 675
7. Chavez, M. D. and Bower, J. D. (1969). Femoro-saphenous arteriovenous shunt for hemodialysis. *Sth. Med. J.*, 62, 345
8. Haimov, M., Burrows, L., Casey, J. D. and Schupak, E. (1973). Vascular access for haemodialysis: Experience with 214 patients special problems and causes for early and late failures. *Proc. E.D.T.A.*, 9, 173
9. Foran, R. F., Golding, A. L., Treiman, R. L. and De Palma, J. R. (1970). Quinton–Scribner cannulas for hemodialysis; review of four years experience. *Calif. Med.*, 112, 8
10. Brescia, M. J., Cimino, J. E., Appel, K. and Hurwich, B. J. (1966). Chronic hemodialysis using venipuncture and a surgically created arteriovenous fistula. *N. Engl. J. Med.*, 275, 1089
11. Haimov, M., Singer, A. and Schupak, E. (1971). Access to blood vessels for hemodialysis: experience with 87 patients on chronic hemodialysis. *Surgery*, 69, 884
12. Tellis, V. A., Veith, F. J., Soberman, R. J., Freed, S. Z. and Gliedman, M. L. (1971). Internal arteriovenous fistulas for hemodialysis. *Surg. Gynecol. Obstet.*, 132, 866
13. Someya, S., Bergan, J. J., Kahan, B. D., Yao, S. T. and Ivanovitch, P. (1976). An upper arm arteriovenous fistula for hemodialysis patients with distal access failures. *Trans. Am. Soc. Artif. Intern. Organs*, 21, 398
14. Beemer, R. K. and Hayes, J. F. (1973). Hemodialysis using a mandril-grown graft. *Trans. Am. Soc. Artif. Intern. Organs*, 19, 43
15. Morgan, A. and Lazarus, M. (1975). Vascular access for dialysis. Technics and results with newer methods. *Am. J. Surg.*, 129, 432
16. May, J., Tiller, D., Johnson, J., Stewart, J. and Shiel, A. G. R. (1969). Saphenous vein arteriovenous fistula in regular dialysis treatment. *N. Engl. J. Med.*, 280, 770

17. Zerbino, V. R. and Tice, D. A. (1973). Successful use of preserved allograft veins for chronic haemodialysis. *Nephron*, **10**, 61

18. Piccone, Jr, V. A., Lee, H., Ramos, S., Ahmed, N., Di Scala, V., Hamanci, M., Piccone III, V. A., Nielsen, E., Le Veen, H. H. and Berger, E. (1975). Preserved allografts of distal saphenous vein for vascular access – an initial experience. *Ann. Surg.*, **182**, 727

19. Bell, P. R. F. and Calman, K. C. (1974). *Surgical Aspects of Haemodialysis*. (Edinburgh and London: Churchill Livingstone)

20. Girardet, R. E., Hackett, R. E., Goodwin, N. J. and Friedman, E. A. (1970). Thirteen months experience with the saphenous vein graft arteriovenous fistula for maintenance hemodialysis. *Trans. Am. Soc. Artif. Intern. Organs*, **16**, 285

21. Santiago-Delphin, E. A., Buselmeier, T. J., Simmons, R. L., Najarian, J. S. and Kjellstrand, C. M. (1972). Modified saphenous vein loop fistula in thigh for chronic hemodialysis. *Surg. Gynecol. Obstet.*, **134**, 835

22. Rosenberg, N., Lord, G. H., Henderson, J., Bothwell, J. W. and Gaughran, E. R. L. (1970). Collagen arterial graft of bovine origin: seven years observations in the dog. *Surgery*, **67**, 951

23. Haimov, M., Burrows, L., Baez, A., Neff, M. and Slifkin, R. (1974). Alternatives for vascular access for hemodialysis: experience with autogenous saphenous vein autografts and bovine heterografts. *Surgery*, **75**, 467

24. Payne, J. E., Chatterjee, S. N., Barbour, B. H. and Berne, T. V. (1974). Vascular access for chronic hemodialysis using modified bovine arterial graft arteriovenous fistula. *Am. J. Surg.*, **128**, 54

25. Vander Werf, B. A. (1973). Bovine graft arteriovenous fistulas for hemodialysis. *Proc. Dial. Transpl. Forum*, **3**, 12

26. Yokoyama, T., Bower, R., Chinitz, J., Schwartz, A. and Schwartz, C. (1974). Experience with 100 arteriografts for maintenance hemodialysis. *Trans. Am. Soc. Artif. Intern. Organs*, **20**, 328

27. Haimov, M. and Jacobson II, J. H. (1974). Experience with the modified bovine arterial heterograft in peripheral vascular reconstruction and vascular access for hemodialysis. *Ann. Surg.*, **180**, 291

28. Merickel, J. H., Anderson, R. C., Knutson, R., Lipschultz, M. L. and Hitchcock, C. R. (1974). Bovine carotid artery shunts in vascular access surgery. *Arch. Surg.*, **109**, 245

29. Rosenberg, N. (1976). The bovine arterial graft and its several applications. *Surg. Gynecol. Obstet.*, **142**, 104

30. De Falco, R. J. (1970). Immunologic studies of untreated and chemically modified bovine carotid arteries. *J. Surg. Res.*, **10**, 95

31. Butt, K. M. H. and Kountz, S. L. (1976). A new vascular access for hemodialysis. The arterial jump graft. *Surgery*, **79**, 476

32. Payne, J. E. and Berne, T. V. (1974). Access to the circulation for haemodialysis. *Med. J. Aust.*, **2**, 667

33. Hermosillo, C. X., Paroa, F., Gordon, H. E. and Wilson, S. E. (1974). Infectability of dacron vs bovine grafts by induced Staphylococcus bacteria. *Surg. Forum*, **25**, 256

34. Jenkins, A. McL. (1976). Gore-Tex: a new prosthesis for vascular access. *Br. Med. J.*, **2**, 280

35. Baker, Jr, L. D., Johnson, J. M. and Goldfarb, D. (1976). Expanded poly-

tetrafluoroethylene (PTFE) subcutaneous arteriovenous conduits: an improved vascular access for chronic hemodialysis. *Trans. Am. Soc. Artif. Intern. Organs*, 22, 382

36. Kaplan, M. S., Mirahmadi, K. S., Winer, R. L., Gorman, J. T., Dabirvaziri, N. and Rosen, S. M. (1976). Comparison of 'PTFE' and bovine grafts for blood access in dialysis patients. *Trans. Am. Soc. Artif. Intern. Organs*, 22, 388

37. Jenkins, A. McL., Picken, C. M. and Halliday, I. M. (1977). Complications following use of expanded polytetrafluoroethylene (Gore-Tex) prostheses for vascular access. *J. R. Coll. Surg. Edin.*, 22, 203

38. Soyer, T., Tempinen, M., Cooper, P., Morton, L. and Eiseman, B. (1972). A new venous prosthesis. *Surgery*, 72, 864

39. Campbell, C. D., Goldfarb, D. and Roe, R. (1975). A small arterial substitute. Expanded microporous polytetralfuoroethylene; patency versus porosity. *Ann. Surg.*, 182, 138

40. Kaegi, A., Pineo, G. F., Shimizu, A., Trivedi, H., Hirsh, J. and Gent, M. (1974). Arteriovenous-shunt thrombosis. *N. Engl. J. Med.*, 290, 304

41. Kaegi, A., Pineo, G. F., Shimizu, A., Trivedi, H., Hirsh, J. and Gent, M. (1975). The role of Sulfinpyrazone in the prevention of arteriovenous shunt thrombosis. *Circulation*, 52, 497

DISCUSSION

J. A. Kanis (Oxford): Antiplatelet drugs were mentioned at the end of the Paper. Mr Jenkins's rate of survival with the Scribner shunt seems to be considerably lower than the experience of many others, where they may survive for many years.

Jenkins: My comment was based on no assessment of figures. I believe it is fairly general experience up to 6 months. There is no formal trial of antiplatelet drugs amongst dialysis patients.

A. Hall (Isle of Man): We have a patient who has had a Scribner shunt for 9 years.

A. M. Martin (Sunderland): Does Mr Jenkins think that there is no longer a need to insert Scribner shunts? It is usually the physicians who do this, and if they lose this skill there may be the not infrequent situation where the patient with acute renal failure requires haemodialysis and ends up with chronic renal failure. If the skill is lost because people such as Mr Jenkins say that the practice is no longer required it will lead to some problems. There will always be a role for a well-inserted Scribner shunt.

Jenkins: I would entirely agree. If the physician is willing to insert the Scribner shunts that is eminently suitable. It depends on the resources of the hospital involved. If someone is willing to be on tap all the time to insert these things then well and good. In Edinburgh the physicians insert a number of Scribners.

Ms Anne T. Lambie (Edinburgh): Perhaps one reason for quoting a 3-month period for the Scribner is that we make no particular attempt to maintain patency for longer periods. They are a transient phenomenon, often abandoned while still working.

Kanis: But for some patients it may be more suitable to have a shunt that can be kept in for many years.

262

J. S. Robson (Edinburgh): Patients make the point that the needle is a major defect – and a defect that could be avoided if we were to get back to the old-fashioned Scribner.

B. H. B. Robinson (Birmingham): Has Mr Jenkins any experience with umbilical vein grafts?

Jenkins: I have not used them. I have tried them experimentally, harvesting our own and putting them into dogs. I know that they are extremely expensive and they do not seem to hold out any great advantage against the other materials that are available.

F. M. Parsons (Leeds): I was a little worried about Mr Jenkins's upper arm Gore-Tex grafts. What rate of flow does he achieve through those grafts? I would suspect that it might produce cardiac embarrassment because the huge lumen of Gor-Tex anastomosed to a very large brachial artery and also to a very large vein. Has he any knowledge of the rate of flow of blood through these?

Jenkins: No. It is very difficult to assess. We have tried out an electromagnetic flowmeter on Gor-Tex but got no recording due to the nature of the conduction of this material.

The graft is only 60 mm internal diameter – no bigger than that. So far we have not seen anyone with cardiac embarrassment indentifiably due to this.

Parsons: I ask because we have put these between femoral artery and femoral vein and have achieved flow rates of between 2 and 2.5 l – which is quite unacceptable to the heart. I would issue a word of caution until flow rates can be given, particularly as a percentage of total cardiac output.

Jenkins: We are cautious about this and we are on the lookout for trouble. They could be banded fairly simply if it should occur.

Parsons: We banded one. It eroded, and that was the end. What material do you use for banding – silk?

Jenkins: I would tend to band with silk. That would be a reasonable thing to do.

Parsons: One of our grafts eroded through the band and that produced an external haemorrhage breaking through the apparently healed incision.

Jenkins: Did the band enter the vascular conduit itself?

Parsons: The whole thing just disrupted.

Miss S. Taber (Cambridge): Can I refer back to the unbilical vein graft. We have one very successful patient in Cambridge. We used 31 cm and it was £250. It is a British-made bovine graft.

Jenkins: We do not use bovine material.

18

The duration of dialysis
A. M. Martin and J. K. Gibbins

18.1   THE CORRELATION BETWEEN BIOCHEMISTRY AND CLINICAL SYMPTOMS

After periods ranging from 4 months to 2 years on 9–10$\frac{1}{2}$ hours haemodialysis weekly, six patients became vaguely unwell over a 2-week period. They developed increasing dyspnoea, anterior chest pain, then pericardial friction. Cardiac tamponade occurred in three cases. The prodromal illness had features not typical of either bronchopneumonia or pulmonary oedema and all had evidence of left ventricular hypertrophy and ischaemia on ECG prior to the illness although only two had previous hypertension. The mean pre-dialysis blood urea at the onset of pericarditis was 39 mmol/l, this being 26% higher than previous levels. These cases represent an incidence of pericarditis of 8% in our dialysis population. Various authors[1] quote an incidence of 10–17% in patients maintained on 'adequate' dialysis.

A 58-year-old mild diabetic was maintained on regular dialysis 10.5 h weekly for 1 year with a mean pre-dialysis blood urea of 33 mmol/l. For a period of 3 months, the first hour of dialysis was replaced by ultrafiltration alone and the pre-dialysis urea levels rose to a mean of 60.1 mmol/l. He was asymptomatic and no pericarditis developed.

These cases are described to illustrate the fact that biochemical status alone does not correlate with clinical symptoms. Perhaps for example in the genesis of pericarditis the state of the left ventricular muscle is of more importance than the blood urea.

We are constantly being confronted with attempts to correlate a great wealth of laboratory data with clinical features in uraemia. The correlations are poor. It is regarded as bad practice to put much emphasis on single case descriptions and instead draw conclusions from large statistically analysed series. This in turn usually provides data inapplicable to the individual patient. Perhaps it is time to pay more attention to the individual patient.

18.2   WORKING GUIDELINES AS TO THE ADEQUACY AND DURATION OF DIALYSIS

Attempts to determine the duration and adequacy of dialysis have been based on inter-related factors. The simplest guide lines are the blood urea, creatinine and potassium concentrations, fluid status and the efficiency of the dialyser. For example, empirically we like the blood urea to be less than 34 mmol/l pre-dialysis. These parameters have been coupled with a consideration of uraemic symptoms, hypertension control and acute dialysis induced symptoms. Tradition and fashion may have had some influence on our use of dialysis and latterly a desire to treat more patients, perhaps with limited facilities, has affected our practice. In our unit, limited facilities stimulated our adoption of a shortened dialysis regime of 3 to $3\frac{1}{2}$ h thrice weekly[2], so that with a staff reduction of 42% and a reduction in renal unit running hours of 40% we were able to increase the number of dialyses by 30%.

18.3 OTHER ELABORATE PARAMETERS

In addition to the simple guidelines I would mention some other elaborate parameters only to discount them as of little practical value in assessing adequacy or duration of dialysis. They include the use of neuro-behavioural probes[3] involving a quantified EEG, photic driving response and continuous performance testing, EMG, motor nerve conduction velocities, the dialysis index[4] which defines middle molecule clearance, kinetic modelling to predict removal rates of urea and creatinine, and finally bone status.

18.4 RANGE OF HAEMODIALYSIS THERAPIES – THE MINIMUM AND OPTIMUM THERAPY

There is no universal optimum duration or type of dialysis. A desire to define this has led to regimens utilizing dialysers with urea clearances ranging from 6 to 180 ml/min at a frequency of one to seven times weekly for dialysis times of 6–168 h per week.

It is probable that the dialysis regime for each patient can be established at two levels. Firstly a type and duration that is the basic minimum which, by controlling dangerous levels of toxins and fluid, keeps the patient alive. Secondly the optimum type and duration which is unique for that patient but variable and results in full rehabilitation. For example, one might say all patients need a minimum of 3–4 h thrice weekly but for optimum therapy this will require variation in duration, ultrafiltration and perhaps even dialysate flow or composition. I think this optimum level can only be arrived at by trial including attending to the patient's own observations. It is possible that an individual adapts in some way to a certain duration and type of dialysis and although they are never normal biochemically, they tolerate regular, similar fluctuations in body chemistry and fluid status.

We have observed one patient who was maintained on an 8h Kiil dialysis thrice weekly and was switched to 3×3 h on a 1.5 m^2 coil. After about 2 weeks he adapted to the therapy in that acute dialysis symptoms were minimal and are now infrequent. He remains well with a blood urea level higher than previously but if we increase the dialysis duration from

3 to 3.5 h the extra half hour induces nausea, vomiting and cramps without any significant ultrafiltration. Initially one was inclined to say this was a psychological reaction to doing an extra half hour. However, I have discounted this and have tried the procedure on several occasions with identical results. We have observed symptoms in one patient on twice weekly 3 h dialysis with a well controlled urea, creatinine and fluid level and little in the way of ultrafiltration required. He regularly developed fatigue and anorexia the day following a dialysis, after a 3 day gap, a phenomenon which did not affect him following the other dialysis of the week. Although urea and creatinine levels were of a similar order it would seem that some change in body chemistry and perhaps metabolism differed between the two dialyses.

On the other hand, two patients were well maintained on 3–3.5 h dialysis thrice weekly for one year. Then without any obvious change in ultrafiltration, dialysate concentration or blood chemistry, they developed regular acute symptoms after about the first hour of every dialysis.

18.5 THE PHYSICAL ADAPTATION TO DIALYSIS

There is no immediate explanation for the occurrences just described and they probably represent two or more different phenomena in the process of physical ADAPTATION to dialysis. I think we are all inclined to explain disturbances on simple grounds and regard most upsets as having similar causes related to excess ultrafiltration, hyponatraemia, exsanguination due to high blood flow rates or hypocalcaemia. However, if we look more carefully at each patient's problems in and around dialysis it is often not possible to relate it to these factors. We may then describe it vaguely as some form of 'disequilibrium' without actually knowing what this means. From the point of view of physical symptoms we can all remember patients who take to dialysis quickly and others who have a prolonged troublesome introduction. It has often been noted that some regular dialysis patients, despite stable biochemistry, require up to 2 years before they are really rehabilitated. There may well be differing rates of metabolic adaptation and once a pattern is set a change may have disturbing effects. It is also possible that intercurrent illness or other disordered function could upset the response to dialysis.

18.6 THE RELATIONSHIP BETWEEN PROTEIN CATABOLISM AND MASS TRANSFER THERAPY

Gotch[6] recently reviewed a series of dialysis–sorbent regimes and analysed the protein catabolic rates in relation to urea removal capacity. He noted that when dialysis was changed from a single pass system to a low volume recirculating system, in addition to a reduction in urea removal there was a reduction in urea production. He suggested that protein catabolic pathways are upset by mass transfer therapy and it is likely that alternative low molecular weight catabolites are formed which are dialysed through standard membranes.

Cambi[7] reviewed the lean body weight of patients treated for up to 9 years by long or short dialysis on free diet. Of his patients 56% commenced treatment above their ideal weight and 44% below. After periods of therapy ranging from 9 months to 9 years on long or short dialysis the body weights were unchanged. It would seem that despite complete symptomatic rehabilitation the patients metabolism may become set at a level consistent with the uraemic and dialysis status but not normal.

It is also probable that the more efficient the dialysis the longer the process of adaptation. Grimsrud[8], using a single pass 100 ml/min dialysate flow, requiring 20–25 l of dialysate for a 3–4 h dialysis thrice weekly with standard dialysers achieved excellent rehabilitation of patients despite high levels of urea and creatinine. Switching from standard high flow to the low flow system resulted in patients having greater ultrafiltration tolerance and a reduction in dialysis related complications.

18.7 CONCLUSION

1. There is probably more uncertainty about the duration and type of dialysis to use now than there was when it was introduced, and there are as many regimens as there are renal units. Perhaps there should be as many regimens as there are patients.

2. Further study of the protein metabolism of the uraemic patient may bring us closer to an understanding of the tolerance and adequacy of dialysis.

3. When Wilhelm Kolff finally perfects the wearable artificial kidney[9] we shall have to think of something other than the duration of dialysis to talk about.

ACKNOWLEDGEMENTS

To Miss J. Davis, Royal Infirmary Sunderland, for constant help and tolerance.

References

1. Hollomby, D., Gonda, A., Morin, J., Long, R. and Dobell, A. R. C., (1975). Uremic pericardial tamponade. *Proc. Dialysis Transplant Forum*, 16–19

2. Martin, A. M., Oduro-Dominah, A., Gibbins, J. K., Devapal, D. and Mitchell, D. C. (1975). Regular short dialysis in end stage renal failure. *Br. Med. J.*, **296**, 758

3. Teschan, P. E., Ginn, H. E., Bourne, J. R., Ward, J. W. and Vaughn, W. K. (1977). Neurobehaviourial probes for adequacy of dialysis. *Trans. Am. Soc. Artif. Intern. Organs.* (In press)

4. Teehan, B., Gracek, E., Heymach, G., Brown, J., Smith, L., Sigler, M., Gilgore, G. and Schleifer, C. (1977). A clinical appraisal of the dialysis index. *Trans. Am. Soc. Artif. Intern. Organs.* (In press)

5. Janssen, H. F., Stanbaugh, G. H. and Holloway, L. S. (1977). Individualised hemodialysis therapy based on Kinetic modelling. *Trans. Am. Soc. Artif. Intern. Organs.* (In press)

6. Gotch, F. (1977). A general review of the progress made in the technical aspects of haemodialysis. Recent Advances in Biochemical Engineering – Technical Aspects of Renal dialysis. University of Newcastle upon Tyne. 4–6 April 1977. (In press)

7. Grimsrud, L., Jørstad, S., Widerøe, T. and Berg, K. J. (1977). Low flow dialysis. *Trans. Am. Soc. Artif. Intern. Organs.* (In press)

8. Cambi, V., Arisl, L., Bignardi, L., Garini, G., Rossi, E., Savazzi, G. and Migone, L. (1975). Short dialysis after 3 years. *Short Dialysis and Uraemic Osteodystrophy.* Opuscula Medico-Technica Lundensia XVI

9. Kolff, W. J. (1977). Honor Lecture. Artificial Organs: Landmarks of the past and prospects of the future. *Trans. Am. Soc. Artifern. Int. Organs.* (In press)

DISCUSSION

Unidentified speaker: What is the attitude of Dr Martin's patients when they find out that other patients spend three to four times as long on the machine at a stretch? Are they pleased or miserable?

Martin: They are quite contented – naturally. We have had patients who have been elsewhere and who have come to us, and they have been exceedingly grateful. It has changed their way of life. There have been spontaneous statements that life is a little more tolerable. I make no exaggerated claims.

A. W. Siemsen (Honolulu): I am curious regarding the patients' reaction when the dialysis regimen is decreased by 30 minutes. This should be done behind a blank wall, with just the tubes coming out through the wall, so that nobody except one person knows how long that patient is on the dialysis.

Martin: That would be essential to really put the finger on whether this was achieving satisfactory dialysis. The problem is that many of our patients control their own dialysis while on the machine. If, for example, they see themselves losing weight they will give themselves saline. I have one particular patient, admittedly he is unique in a group of about 30 patients, who knows when the 3 hours are up even if he cannot see the clock. He knows things are happening and he must stop, and he will look at his weight, and it has not changed.

J. S. Robson (Edinburgh): Surely there are more patients who know when 5 hours are up. I suspect that a number of patients who go to 5 hours then experience cramp, or discomfort, and learn to recognize it.

Martin: Yes. It is quite common. But can one put a finger on why they have cramp?

Robson: No.

J. A. Kanis (Oxford): There are some animal models for the adaptation of protein metabolism that lend credibility to Dr Martin's suggestions. The first is the adaptation of protein metabolism that occurs in the brown bear hibernating in winter.

The other is some fascinating observations presented to the European Society for Clinical Investigation in 1976 whereby uretus transplanted in the peritoneum resulted in a longer survival of uraemic rats than nephrectomized rats maintained on the same fluid and electrolyte regime[1]. The difference in survival was very marked.

Martin: It would be a very difficult study in the human.

R. Ahmad (Liverpool): Referring to the patient who develops a syndrome after 3 hours, surely he has a positive membrane pressure. Even if there is no dialysate pressure on the machine, he is still ultrafiltrating.

Dr Martin hit the nail on the head. All patients are different and dialysis should be tailor-made for every individual. My patients range from 9 or 10 hours dialysis a week to as much as 24 hours a week. It is connected with the age, sex and muscle mass of the patient, perhaps even the diagnosis, and many other factors.

Martin: Whatever the cause, there would seem to be a variation in how much dialysis is necessary.

Ahmad: I find it increasingly hard to accept $3\frac{1}{2}$ hours of dialysis for every Tom, Dick and Harry. A paper was recently published on someone who started dialysing $3\frac{1}{2}$ hours three times a week and from 16 patients there were four deaths in the first 6 weeks.

Martin: It amounts to how low one can go before one worries.

Ahmad: It has to be determined for the individual patient.

A. C. Kennedy (Glasgow): There are tremendous variations in how much uraemia a patient can stand. We have all seen patients with uraemia who have been remarkably fit, going about a job, and so on, with very high serum creatinines, low haemoglobins, etc. and others who are sick and who present to the doctor as being sick. There is a tremendous difference in acceptability of uraemia.

Robson: Has Dr Martin any advice on how to proceed to find out how much treatment to give to individual patients?

Kennedy: We should go different ways and frequently compare results. It is important for us not to get preset ideas that we must have X or Y. We really do not know. There is need for more flexibility and different approaches.

Robson: But to take one approach and to stick to it for 6 months or 9 months and then change is to go away from individualization because a unit may have a hundred patients.

Kennedy: Even within that.

Ms Anne T. Lambie (Edinburgh): What criteria would Professor Kennedy use in comparing results?

Kennedy: I would have a list of things that I think are very bad to have, such as haemorrhagic pericarditis, uncontrollable hypertension, symptomatic bone disease and so on. I published an article several years ago[2] on a scoring system whereby patients got more adverse points if they developed certain nasty things, or things that I thought were nasty, and the one with the lowest total was doing best. The theme was not taken up. Perhaps there is a need for groups in a country, like the UK, to try to get some agreement and measure a certain number of things subsequently comparing them on a quantitative basis.

Martin: In the North-East (England) we have an ongoing MRC trial comparing acute dialysis symptoms and long-term effects in three groups of patients: home dialysis patients who are entirely on Meltec dialysers, hospital dialysis patients in Newcastle using the polyacrylonitrile dialyser, and our own. My patients have the shortest dialysis time. Information is coming in but the long-term information will be of the utmost value. However, I suspect that we still have not yet found the right things to measure.

Miss Mary E. Selsby (London): What weight gain do Dr Martin's patients have between dialysis?

Martin: From 1 to 1.5 and sometimes 2 kg, with $3-3\frac{1}{2}$ h dialysis thrice a week. We had one patient who was on twice a week, but I have just switched him simply because of the symptom that I described, namely that after a long gap he did not feel good. Now he feels fantastic, yet I have made no difference to his chemistry.

Mrs M. Brown (Manchester): What are the average haemoglobin levels of these patients on short-hour dialysis?

Martin: Overall it is probably 7–8 g/dl.

M. K. Ward (Newcastle-upon-Tyne): There is no real difference between the other two groups in the comparison. The polyacrylonitrile patients are slightly better but this is not yet statistically significant.

Unidentified speaker: We have not heard much about dietary control, or about the heparin control of the patients for the short duration in view of the pericarditis.

Martin: None of our patients are on protein restriction. We are only careful about high potassium intake and fluid. Whether they are on fluid control depends on whether they are making urine. The majority are not. The majority of the patients would be on 750 ml/24 h. The majority of creatinine clearances are zero, although one or two have 2 or 3 ml/minute.

The quantity of heparin used is less than that given for long dialysis and is given as a single bolus injection at the beginning of treatment.

References

1. Schuck, O., Skopkova, J. and Gort, J. (1976). The 'excretory intelligence' of the gut in rats without renal excretion. Abstracts of European Society for Clinical Investigation, no. 194.
2. Kennedy, A. C., Lindsay, R. M., Murphy, A. V., Allison, M. E. M., McLeod, O. (1971). A scoring system for assessing patients on regular dialysis. *Lancet*, i, 701

CONCLUSIONS
A. C. Kennedy

This symposium has been made possible by the generosity and sponsorship of Travenol Laboratories and I am sure that you would wish me to express on your behalf our gratitude to them, and in particular our gratitude to the organizer, Mr Peter Irving. I also know that he would wish me to comment on the help that he received from the committee, Deirdre Jones, John Anderton and Frank Parsons, for the assistance that they gave him. I know that Travenol would be interested in having reactions as to how valuable the Symposium has been, on whether the content of the programme was right, and on the content of the individual papers, bearing in mind the mixed nature of the audience. These comments can either be passed on verbally, when meeting people from Travenol, or they can be sent in in writing.

I shall now use the chairman's privilege to make some remarks that seem to me appropriate.

Speaking as a clinician I think we have had a series of balanced accounts and appraisals of various facets of current practice in the UK. This is always useful. It is a form of painless postgraduate instruction that is very good for clinicians from time to time. It is very useful to realize that the problems I have in my unit are the same problems that everybody else has, and that there is no mysterious magic thing that I should be doing or should have started to do 6 months ago. From the clinician's point of view it was a success.

For the nursing staff, the technical staff, and the other staff relating to dialysis units, I would hope that taken as a whole there was enough in the Symposium to have given them useful guidance on various aspects of practical management. If at times they perhaps felt that the content of the occasional paper had rather too much actual physiology or something that was perhaps not of immediate interest or relevance to them, they should bear with us in this. It is useful for them to understand the complexities that underline these problems and why some of these problems are so difficult to solve.

For those from the Department of Health, the Ministry, in the audience I think that a very clear message came across – a very clear picture of hardworking units, underfinanced. I would hope that the message is taken back, digested and analysed – and even more hopefully, acted on.

Finally, for everyone – doctors, nurses, technical staff, etc., and including the commercial people themselves – there were two clear-cut benefits. First there was the opportunity to meet and make contact with people from other units and related disciplines. This is always enormously valuable. Secondly, we have had the opportunity to hear two very moving but very modest accounts of actually living with renal failure from Mr Baillie and from Dr Henry. Their papers were an inspiration to us all.

Thank you very much.

Index